MW01279882

Decisions to Make

Paths to Take

Decisions to Make
Paths to Take

A Guide for Caregivers

Joy Pelzmann, Ph.D. and Myrna Rosoff, J.D.

Decision Press

Boynton Beach, FL 33474

DECISION PRESS
P.O. Box 741254
BOYNTON BEACH, FL 33474-1254

Printed in the United States of America

Published by Decision Press

P.O. Box 741254, Boynton Beach, FL 33474-1254

Library of Congress Catalog Number 97-94562

ISBN 0-9661189-0-1

With the exception of "Together At Last" and "New Thresholds", all
anecdotes in this book are fictional. Names, characters, places and
incidents are the product of the authors' imagination. Any resemblance
to actual persons, living or dead, events or locales, is entirely
coincidental.

First Printing

Authors: Joy Pelzmann, Ph.D. and Myrna Rosoff. J.D.

Cover Artist: Matthew Cohen
Portrait Photography: Frank Donnino
Sentinel Printing, St. Cloud, MN

This book is dedicated to children,

spouses, friends and all those who care

for all those who need care.

Let the words of my mouth

and the meditation of my heart

be acceptable in thy sight...

Psalm XIX, 14

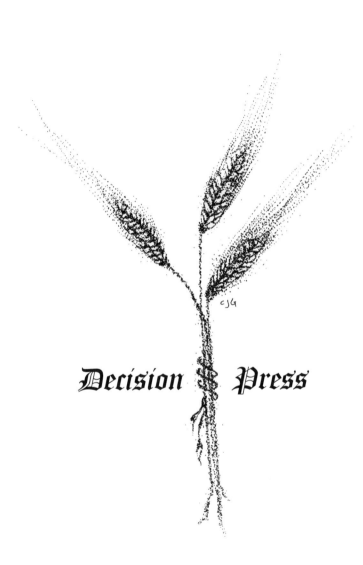

Decision ☙ Press

Table of Contents

Do not delay until the time feels right, but begin your healing now. Do not replicate the choices of the past in the behaviors of the present.

PREFACE

This is a book that came into being of its own
volition, out of the pain and experience, and sometimes,
out of the joy, that each of us had caring for our parents.
The surprises of the journey, and our own opportunity to
evolve in this process, encouraged us to explore more
fully the demands of our new and growing role of
caregiver, and once we understood our function, to
determine how to combine this with an already busy life.
While we grappled with the practicalities, there were also
emotional, philosophical and spiritual problems to which
we found no easy answers elsewhere. Yet it was these very
answers that we felt would give us the strength we needed
most in these difficult and uncertain times.

If there is a basic premise to this book, it is that
reconciliation and renewal are possible when one acts
with consciousness and intent to resolve the unfinished
business of lifelong relationships. With increased
awareness, disappointment and dread can be supplanted
by appreciation for each day, and for each other. It is our
hope that this book will offer both strategies and support
as you pursue your answers.

There may be concepts put forward here that are foreign to you, or that represent a point of view you may have ignored or previously rejected. If God has not been part of your world view, this is an opportunity to examine and explore new and enriching possibilities. This certainly has been our experience, one that is beyond all that we might have imagined.

This book not only came out of our experience with family members, it arose out of our personal practice as well. Students of t'ai chi and meditation, we have sought stillness to find understanding, suspending activity to direct our awareness inward. In the openness of our meditations, information was given which we share with you now. As you will see throughout the book, the format is one of questions and answers, a format which appealed to both of us, educated as we were in traditional professions. And so it happened that a retired attorney framed these questions while a retired psychology professor sat in meditation awaiting for responses to be given. We have no desire to give further explanation for this process, but it is heartfelt and meaningful, and we find both comfort and wisdom in the words presented. We hope you read them with the same openness, and derive benefit in the understanding that is offered.

To the parent, we say that this is the time to value your child, to renew bridges of affection and understanding, and seek peace of mind. To the parent, the child remains the child, no matter how old. To the child, we present the belief that with consciousness and intent, it is possible to reach a greater understanding and resolution of the intimate connection between parent and child. There lies before you discovery of the parent you always hoped to have, or perhaps had, and have long since tucked away in your memory. Both of you have the opportunity to explore a complicated, challenging phase of existence, the end of life, and the loss of all that is familiar, and to do it as a shared journey rather than an isolated experience, an opportunity to explore and expand rather than suffer alone in the wilderness. To husbands and wives, while the intimacy is of later origin and created out of different needs, the discoveries and rewards can be equally powerful.

As you venture forth with us, a meditation is offered to help you participate in this discovery. Read this and let the intent travel with you throughout your journey.

May my heart inform my mind,

May the words I read be shaped by the
      compassion I carry within.

May God's grace enter this space with me.

May I offer compassion to others as I
      wish it offered to me.

Listen to your heart. This is a Path that only you can walk and choices only you can make. The wisdom required to understand is already present. Trust your senses and your heart's choices. There are no others.

CHAPTER I

INTRODUCTION

Life is filled with changes and challenges and
increased longevity carries with it a host of additional
ones. Changes of form, changes of expectation and the
gradual erosion of energy are challenges that everyone
faces. Not only must people deal with their own aging, but
many adults struggle with the problems of the aging of
another, for increasingly large numbers will be
responsible for the care of an elderly person at some point
in life.

You are reading this book, so you acknowledge
your involvement with this major responsibility, or sacred
obligation, depending on your point of view. Probably you
are now helping and guiding another person through the
final stages of their life, sometimes willingly, sometimes
grudgingly. No matter your disposition, various aspects of
another person's welfare are in your hands. For both of
you, this can move out of the realm of drudgery and
burden to become a most rewarding experience. The
amount of time you expend and the degree of

responsibility you assume will vary depending on living arrangements, the closeness of relationship, geography, the availability of others to share the tasks, and even financial resources. For the "nuts and bolts" of the job you face, we have included an appendix of agencies that can help you locate the resources you need on both local and national levels. There is no question that the practical concerns of housing and care are pressing, but it is the problems of heart, soul, and psyche that will probably cause you the most pain. This book is intended to help provide you with the emotional guidance and spiritual direction to live this opportunity, rather than just get through it. While recognizing that the people most frequently involved in caregiving are usually children and spouses, the intent and application of this book is universal. In fact, we are always another's keeper, just as they serve as ours. We are all one.

The coming chapters offer guidelines and answers to many of the painful questions that arise as you enter this new role. We all try to fulfill our duty; we do what we have to do, and we do it as best we can. Here, however, it is our intent to offer you the tools to turn duty into a service of love, offered from a loving heart, presenting opportunities for emotional and spiritual growth, and even laughter. We also wish to help you identify difficulties that exist now, unrecognized perhaps, but felt as disquiet and doubt, problems which impede you on your path to awareness.

This book taken as a whole provides an overview of the life process as life ends. It is best to read it slowly, and then reflect, before going on. Take a moment to ask yourself, "Does this apply to me? Is this how I am feeling?" These are some of the questions for you to reflect upon or share. The book lends itself to discussion with friends and family as you find further questions and issues brought to mind. You might want to start by scanning the table of contents, which lists the questions most people struggle with at this time. Turn to the question that seems most compelling and read the answer, then give yourself a chance to absorb the material. Do not worry about reading in order, but let your heart lead you. At some later point in time you may wish to go back and read from the beginning in an orderly fashion, but not just yet. The material is very intense, offered with love, but with little attempt made to soften the impact of the words. The guides who offer this information are gentle and compassionate and offer you truth, but this truth can be challenging as well as comforting. They bring you an opportunity to grow in wisdom, not escape in easy platitudes. It is important that you read with an open mind and heart. Allow yourself to experience rather than judge this information.

Throughout the book you will find meditations which are offered as a formal approach to gain calm, inner quiet and understanding. Through meditation we achieve awareness, which is a way of viewing life's experience with alertness and sensitivity to the emotional climate of the moment. Meditations can be focused, and some of the meditations offered are so directed. Others can invited deep contemplation or even simple awareness. While suggestions are offered as to how the meditations may best serve you, they are yours to bring home to your heart. In a very real sense this entire book is a meditation on the impermanence, change and transcendence of life. We hope it will provide reassurance, comfort and joy where none may have been thought possible.

Tend to those who need you; steady your heart and bury your past; your future need not repeat your history. Good outcomes may arise from bad beginnings. Transcend your fears and feel the Lord protecting and comforting always.

CHAPTER II

BETWEEN PARENT AND CHILD

In an ideal world, and under the best of circumstances, parents would approach the end of their life's journey surrounded by loving family willing and able to take over and care for them. Children would know and respect the wishes of the parent, finances would be provided, and intimate and warm communication would be frequent. But sadly, this is not a perfect world, and for most of us, parents and children alike, life is spent dealing with the mundane and many responsibilities of each moment, rather than building the deep understanding and open communication needed under the most challenging circumstances.

In a society such as this one, where parents may live at some distance from their children, estrangement can be as much a matter of geography as it is of interpersonal obstacles. Parents generally have friendship networks separate from their children, and children often develop independent lives in other cities. Family members can become virtual strangers, corresponding by card, an occasional gift, and awkward phone calls at scheduled times. We believe family relationships are far too important to exist in this fashion. Fortunately, the situation is easily improved, requiring only awareness and the willingness to share lives. It is never too early to begin to create a meaningful connection with parents, nor is it ever too late. The time to begin is the moment you realize the situation is worth changing. There is much to be gained in knowing your parent, and much to be learned about who you are. It is always valuable for your parent to know who you have become. Without these vital connections, distance through both time and geography can lead to separation and even distrust.

1.   How does one go about establishing trust so late in life?

There are many places where trust can be developed between parent and child. It might be wise to begin with areas where trust is easiest, and confidence of success greatest. This means it is probably unwise to begin work on trust around issues of money. While money may be a private and sensitive topic for most people, it is even more difficult to address this issue with children. Money may even be the last arena in which parents can exercise control. In the worst of cases sharing financial matters makes them vulnerable to exploitation. Even without that fear, they are vulnerable to your criticism spoken or implied, as it pertains to their performance in a world where success is measured largely in material resources. Your success, too, may be called into question as your parent assumes a critical defensive posture. Seeking to build trust, you must always remember this is not a time for airing old grievances, or for a clash of philosophies, but a time to create bridges of awareness and affection. You may be fortunate and find these connections are still there, but little used or understood. On the other hand, paths separated by distance, generations and activities, may result in connections that are less intimate than those you experienced in childhood.

No matter how cordial before, as events change and difficulties emerge in the life of your parents, your relationship with them may take on a new dimension. Here at last is an opportunity to recreate, or even create for the first time, a richer, more meaningful relationship between the two of you.

2.   You have said money is a poor place to begin. What is a better place to build trust?

Trust is best built in the context of lovingkindness, the realization that we are all connected, an awareness that all are linked by memories, caring and life itself. It is more readily built in the leisurely connection of caring moments, rather than in a brief, intense attachment that springs into being next to the hospital bed. In reality, there may not be time to build this trust, connection and the companionable openness you desire, but the opportunity awaits if you wish it to be so.

One of the best ways to begin is with things you both enjoy. In young adulthood, the relationship between parent and child is about defining differences, not recognizing similarities. In an effort to become an individual, separation and individuality are emphasized. How often have you reflected on the many ways you are not like your parent, rather than the ways in which you are similar? Now begin with the similarities, those many positive qualities that join you together. As you think and speak of these, let a smile and a sense of wonder greet even those traits you would prefer not to have in common. As connection builds, you create a field where bonds of friendship, interdependence and trust can develop.

It is also true that issues of trust are seldom addressed in advance of need, and may surface for the first time in a crisis. At such a time, the parent may have no alternative but to trust the child, because they cannot manage the situation themselves. This is a sacred time, for trust offered and accepted is always a powerful spiritual transaction, but this is only the beginning, for social and legal considerations create a situation far more complicated. Ideally, circumstances would provide an easy transfer of responsibility from one to another, and the trust would be so broad, so wide, and so beautifully woven, no difficulties would arise. In reality, trust most likely is offered piecemeal. It will be a patchwork of the right to make health decisions, but not necessarily the right to sign a check; or the right to take care of the apartment, but not necessarily the right to help decide where a parent will live; or some other combination of financial, emotional and practical responsibilities. Each of these will require different strategies for management and provide unique challenges.

Trust is best built out of affection and respect. If you cannot enter your parent's space with respect in your heart for the soul they are, trust cannot be established. As a child wishing to build trust with a parent, it might be helpful to meditate at the outset, seeking the ability to remain open, loving and compassionate in this interaction, creating a climate in which trust can grow. Perhaps this meditation will prove helpful.

Meditation

This is a time to pause in quiet, if possible in seclusion and to take a few moments to breathe regularly and deeply. Now read the following words softly to yourself a few times, and allow the calm of the words to enter your soul.

Give me the strength to be someone whom
I do not often see,

To allow myself the openness which will
permit me to be the person I have
always wanted to be toward my parent.

Let me sit at their feet and feel the light of
love encircle us both.

3.   **In the best of circumstances, there would be ample time to develop trust. When crisis hits, time is a luxury. Is there any choice but to speak bluntly of finances and basic needs?**

This is a valid point. More often than not, little is known and less is planned. First, be mindful that the moment a crisis occurs is not a time for blame and recrimination. If both parents are alive, the parent who is not in active crisis may feel great shame or embarrassment that they have not handled things better up to this point and in preparation for it. Their plans certainly did not include living their lives in anticipation that someday they would be held accountable by their children for their lack of foresight. You may be tempted to return the blame and condemnation you have received from them during your life. There may be momentary satisfaction in this, but little is to be gained, and it is the critical needs of this moment that must be addressed.

Encouraging your parent to make decisions in situations they have previously avoided may be the most difficult aspect of your intervention. Frustrations mount and focus may be lost. The issue is not so much, "Who is in charge?" and "Who is making the decisions?", but rather the issue is how to engage in this difficult process of choices and outcomes as humanely as possible.

4.   **How is the parent-child relationship reshaped in this time of shifting needs and abilities?**

Let us begin by stating that the parent is never the child, and the child is never the parent. In this lifetime, it is the parent who has accepted the responsibility to raise and nurture the child from helpless dependency to adulthood and independence. It is true that when physical abilities change or intellectual functions diminish, it is easy to see your parent as childlike. Remember, it is their body, it is their ego that is altered, but not their soul. This is still the soul that accepted responsibility for you, their child, and this relationship of parent and child is immutable. Though the specific tasks of the role of each may vary across time, the relationship is never altered. Regardless of your concerns, it is wise at all times to respect the decisions of your parent.

Linking Generations

It happened every year, and Frances didn't like it one bit. Sooner rather than later, her son would get her alone during his annual visit and start asking her questions about her money. Yes, Scott was a good provider for his family, but the way they spent money, how could he ever understand what it meant to live on a counted dollar. He meant well, but she knew he would tell her to sell the stock her husband had bought before his death, and tell her she kept too much money in checking, and he could get a better return on her money with little risk. What did he know about risk? She went to work so he could go to a good college, and she went back to work when she was in her fifties and her husband's business failed. Between social security, the few investments and savings, she got along just fine. She didn't need her son's pity; she didn't need him second guessing what she and her husband had done with their lives. Much better that he believe she really didn't like to travel, rather than know she could not afford it.

Three months later Scott was back visiting Frances, this time without the family. Frances knew she was lucky; the effects of the stroke had mostly disappeared, but she still had trouble remembering things. It was time to let go of her pride and have Scott help handle her affairs. She had a booklet from AARP that set out all the things to be dealt with, and she was determined to see it through, power of attorney, bank accounts, everything, including what she wanted done if she got sick again.

Scott sat quietly, looking at Frances and seeing the frail woman who now dwelled inside her still considerable size. In spite of the downward pull of her mouth and the slurred speech, her performance was intelligent and impressive. More than that, as it became apparent to him just how little his Mom and Dad had lived on, he was filled with admiration for their unfailing optimism and support of his goals. From

a heart filled with love, he complimented her on
her acumen and judgment, and assured her that
he would respect all her wishes. They passed the
next two days in happy reminiscence, in laughter
and in tears, closer than they had ever been
before, or perhaps just appreciating each other
more.

Do not pull yourself away, but allow the moments to seize you. Trust your heart's strength; it will endure.

CHAPTER III

LOVE AND COMPASSION

It is easy to speak of respect, for respect is less intimate than love, and therefore frequently easier to offer as well as receive. To love, on the other hand, is to rely on well known habits that make another endearing. The task that then emerges is how to continue loving someone when these familiar qualities are gone, and instead of the parent of your memories you face a frightened stranger. Your sense of loss is immediate, and the desire to turn away, to flee, is not uncommon. The greatest gift in this situation is compassion, compassion both for you and for your loved one. Forget your defenses and open your heart. To recognize another's distress and be moved to help rather than pity, is a work that heals all engaged in the endeavor.

5. **How is it possible to love a parent when all that remains is the recollection of who they used to be?**

Be aware that love is delivered for the soul that continues even in the diminished person of the present. You have unlimited quantities of love to offer and to receive, and never will it be needed more than now. Time is finite, and there is finite willingness and opportunity to do for another, but the capacity to send love is infinite. There is no way to deplete the love that wells within when it is offered to others. This concept may seem unrealistic, but the very act of opening your heart to others fills you more completely than you might ever have imagined.

No doubt, this is a difficult and troubling time, probably the most troubling aspect of life's journey. Yet the relationship between parents and children is a wonderful opportunity to work on developing compassion, forgiveness, and understanding. To work on being fully present in each moment is to work on love, and on opening your heart to the full intensity of life's experience.

6.   As the body deteriorates, the elderly person asks, "How can I be loveable in this form, as I am now?"

It is sad that so much attention is paid to something with so little meaning as the external appearance of form. The love that comes from love of someone's form, or their beauty, wit, or even wisdom, is superficial compared to the deep and enduring connection that comes from the love of heart to heart, and soul to soul. Aging flesh does not preclude the opportunity for joy. It may serve as an excuse for no longer hoping to find joy, but there is always space in the heart for love, and there is always space in the heart of others to love in return. Do not let the illusion of an aging or frail body hide this very profound truth.

7.   But if you don't love someone for the face they present to the world, or for the mind that filters the world, what do you love?

Love is not about form. It is very much a connection like that of molecules meeting. The fit is good, the polarities are joined, and the connection has meaning. Your assumption that connection rests on the body is made out of habit. Actually, it is the soul hearing the echo response from another that creates love of the highest level. This does not denigrate other forms of love, it merely means that the purest love is always available, even if the ordinary cues of social or erotic love are not present. You will note as you look at the most aged of the aged, that they still have the capacity to love and form deep emotional bonds with one another. It is not that they are too foolish to understand otherwise. It is that they are too wise to neglect it. Do not miss the wisdom that is offered and accept it for the gift it is.

8.   We are instructed to find compassionate connections. How is this done?

First, you must learn to love yourself. This does not mean drawing up a list of your good points and your flaws, nor does it mean engaging in self-indulgence.

Loving yourself means appreciating that core of goodness that resides in each of you and is called soul. Accept who you are, a person worth loving. It is only when you feel that you are worth loving that you are capable of offering love from the heart instead of the mind.

The difference between love from the heart and love from the mind is clear. Love offered from the heart is unconditional, unmeasured, and expects nothing in return. Love offered from the mind also may be offered fully, but it is offered in the hope that something will be returned for its expression. This return may be love, support, gratitude, respect, money or any other form of gratification. When love goes through the mind instead of the heart, it is subject to distortion. The desires of the giver taint the love that is given.

These ideas are important, but so are the everyday enactments. There are many mundane ways in which compassionate connections can be made. Perhaps the easiest is sharing food, breaking bread together. When life feels its bleakest, the only taste that may remain is for the very sweetest in life. So it may be candy you share, or ice cream, or a flavorful meal, easy to consume, not large, but kindly delivered. The familiar foods of childhood often are most effective.

Remember, first you must love yourself in your heart, then move out from your heart, almost indiscriminately, offering love to others as it is offered through God's compassion to you. As you send it out, you will find the world radiates back vitality and love in return, and a network of loving thoughts and kindness is constructed.

9. It seems strange to speak of food at this time. Why do you stress its importance?

The act of deciding to eat, the communal act of sharing food, and the meaning of nourishment for the body are profoundly significant and often neglected, particularly when other issues compete for attention. Although much attention is placed on the act of eating, there is little awareness of the deep and abiding connections this act provides. It is a perfect opportunity for awareness, an opportunity to respect and fulfill the preferences of one whose world is greatly restricted. Shared meals feed far more than the body, they can feed the soul as well. Meals surrounded with prayer can be most meaningful, and individuals who give thanks at mealtimes gain much spiritually out of their recognition of the intimate connection of all on the earth, and in the heavens.

10. Please help us to understand compassion.

You must discover your heart's space. This receives little attention in a lifetime where the desire to protect yourself against injury often is far greater than the desire to open to compassion and awareness. Consequently, many individuals, protecting themselves from pain, have gone long years without opening their heart, Yet it is this

open heart that allows compassion to be offered to
yourself and to others.

It is difficult in this secular society to speak of
opening the heart to God's wishes, or even to that still,
small voice within. It is far easier to maintain a facade
and habit of protection. However, if you are to join in life's
adventure, first open your heart without fear, whether it is
opened to sorrow or to joy. With this true awareness
grows and the soul is allowed to expand until it fills the
universe.

We know it is not an easy task to love yourself,
especially when you are consumed with panic, fear,
anger, and confusion. When you are first faced with a
parent or spouse in failing health, the natural thoughts
are often of the impact this will have on your life, not on
the opportunities it can offer to both of you. At the same
time, do not feel disloyal or unworthy if you harbor a
secret hope that you will now finally resolve a conflict,
or earn your parent's love or appreciation. It is normal
and acceptable to feel deeply mixed and conflicted
emotions at this time, and the initial reaction is shock
that your life can so abruptly change forever. Suddenly
dropped into new territory, you are unfamiliar with what
is required of you, and your fears may fill you with
foreboding. Contrary to these fears, there is no long,
dark tunnel; there is only this decision, this action, to
be addressed now, at this moment.

In the first flush of this crisis, the desire is to do
much and through your action erase the impact of all

that has changed. Instead, this is the time to take a deep breath, and quiet your mind. Worries and concerns will wait while you take care of yourself. Nurture yourself and have confidence that you will get through this difficult passage as you have through others. Seek help from those who surround you, from professionals, from family and friends, and if you are comfortable in doing so, from God.

More Than Getting By
With Laughter

They have been inseparable ever since Ed moved into Fairwood Manor six months ago. Ellie, a resident for the past year and a half, liked his sense of humor, and took him under her wing. She even changed her table in the dining room so they could eat together. Now there was a table for six, and the tablemates could usually be counted on for some good laughs. Lately, though, Ed had been annoying Ellie with his constant complaining. Not that he didn't have cause to complain. Heck, they were all in pain. At their stage of life, she liked to say, you either had pain or you were dead and too dumb to lay down. She loved him, but as Ed started up again with, "I'm in pain. So much pain. I don't know what to do." She responded conversationally, "Drop dead." Ed paused, nodded his head up and down. "You know," he said, "that's not a bad idea. Maybe I will." His eyes sparkled as Ellie whooped with laughter, soon joined by everyone around them.

More Than Getting By
With Love

His back is so badly bowed his chin rests on his chest, and he is forced to twist his head upward to see who is talking to him. His walking is a little off balance because of his posture, but he is helped by the tall woman at his side, whose arm is linked through his. They are sweethearts, courtly and serious. They always sit on the same sofa in the lobby, near the center of the large room, where the entertainers set up their instruments. As the music begins, an angry woman comes over to them, and begins to shout and pummel him over some imagined slight. His sweetheart, without hesitation, rises and joins battle. The agitated woman pushes her and breaks her beads before being subdued. In return, she collects some good shoves, and has her hair pulled. As the women are separated, there is a final round of name calling. Everyone is astir and invigorated by the display of passion. Another resident who wanted to intervene is patiently counseled by her neighbors not to get involved. The sweethearts settle back down on "their" sofa.

Later the couple gets up to dance. With his bent posture, she towers a head taller than he. She wraps him in her arms, his head nestled on her chest, and they sway to the music. I look at them and wonder if I am the only one moved to tears by the beauty of their loving connection.

CHAPTER IV

THE REALITY OF AGING

Aging is a gradual, almost imperceptible process. Slowly your parent yields to the inroads of time and becomes increasingly dependent. As the years pass, adjustments must be made emotionally, as well as physically, and you, the child become engaged in a new and far more involved role than you have had with your parent previously. Crisis occurs and stabilizes, and a new routine is established as you begin to assume the role of caregiver. In the midst of all these adjustments, you look at your parent and struggle to recognize the person they have become, and to find your place in this changed reality. Now is the time to reflect on what has come to pass, to ask the questions that seem to have no answer.

11. How can I comfort and care for this parent who is now a stranger to me?

You speak of a stranger, yet this is no stranger. In spite of physical or mental changes, the soul of your parent is unchanged. Move beyond the usual reactions, move beyond the body and its infirmities and look for understanding and connection on a higher plane. Begin to really see your parent. This is easily said in the abstract, but what can you do? First, you must come to terms with the fact that you, too, will walk this long path. Look closely in your mirror, you will find that without realizing it you have become the replacement for that young, vibrant, effective parent of your memory. Clearly, some of your despair at this time relates as much to the inevitability of your own aging and decrepitude as to the losses your parent suffers. Until you truly integrate and accept your position on the wheel of time, you will be tempted to transform your personal anxiety and concern into distress regarding your parent. Only if you to come to terms with your own changes, and the inevitability of your own death, will you be free to join your parent in a transformed relationship, a partnership of sorts. Viewpoints, once opposing and antagonistic, become merely generational as you both engage in this shared exploration. Your parent, though frail, may be more fully available and present than they have been before. This is an opportunity to be taken, a door to be opened. It is God's will that you share this journey together.

12.　And for the parent, is a similar struggle unfolding, with the question instead being, "What has happened to my body?"

Living on the physical plane, it is only natural that losses be seen as final. But in truth there is a cycle to life. When you ride in the car, and you turn from one street onto another, do you ask the person on the seat next to you, "Where did Main Street go now that we are on Oak Street?" No, of course not, because you know full well that although you are present at one place, the other still exists. It exists in the reality you understand because you have been able to go back and forth many times. It is no different in life, though perhaps harder to accept this truth. At the end of this physical lifetime, it seems everything is past and nothing is ahead. This is merely the vantage at this time, a vantage that can be changed, and will be changed time and time again.

We are aware that this may not be a satisfactory example, but life does go on. It is experienced through a sequence of opportunities and exchanges, in which you have both learned lessons and given them. There are many paths you have not taken, and to some, at the end, it may seem there are more regrets than pleasures recalled. Yet the experiences of this lifetime have brought you to this point. You have created connections, shared with others, and provided untold impact on people you cannot even imagine, let alone recollect. Like a pebble falling into a still pond, the ripples have spread far and wide. It would be wonderful if you could be aware of the effect you have had on others, but rest assured that many have felt your presence and remember you with kindness.

13.   How do we approach the many changes and what can we learn from them?

It is true many changes occur, but without these changes and what seem like losses, it would be difficult

for most people to realize that the body has little real
meaning. It is one thing to say change is a natural
process, but quite another to experience how much it
does matter when the body fails to meet your
expectations, no matter how modest these may have
become. This process, a contraction of sorts, is
unpleasant and unrelenting, but necessary, for it begins
the shift from the busy world of doing into the inner
world of knowing. "Knowing what?" you may ask.
Knowing that you are merely travelers through this world.
Deep down you always knew this road awaited you, you
just never acknowledged that you would reach this
corner. It is a difficult task to face diminished abilities, an
unpleasant future beyond contemplation. It is further
compounded by your parent's realization that each falling
away, each letting go, imposes a burden on someone else,
most likely someone they love. This is hardest of all for
those who have struggled their entire lives to be self-
sufficient and never to be a burden to their children. It is
hard to need help, and even harder to accept help. It may
be easier to send others away, reject them, or impart
unkind motives onto their good intentions, as a way of
keeping oneself from being overwhelmed by the intense
feelings of this time.

14.   How do both parent and child cope with this new reality?

The quandry created by these changes can be
managed in several ways. On the most practical level, do
all you can to help your parent maintain a level of
independence which is consistent with their ability at
this time. You might do this by creating an opportunity to

make choices, however small, in many situations, including the difficult ones. For you, the child, it is now time to face the truth that your parent needs your help, just as you one day may need the help of your children or friends. For the parent, relax and recognize that what is being done for you is done for you in love. Dealing with these changes of the body is part of life's work, a challenge, but a manageable one.

As poor a vessel as the body may seem, the soul resides in the body for a reason. This particular body holds some quality essential to you and how you define yourself, and it is such qualities that comprise the ego. These qualities may be beauty, intelligence, the ability to take care of others, or strength, for example. This is central to how you see yourself, and it is this vision of yourself that forms the basis of ego. Regardless of these basic descriptors of ego and self, change will occur. The strong man will grow less strong. The mother will be less able to feed the many, and the mind may lose its agility and retentiveness. Beauty, too, fades with age. These are great gifts and there is sadness as they are taken away, but be assured, this is not a tragic thing. Your greatest asset is not a chance accident of genetics, but rather your intrinsic worth rests in your soul. If you allow yourself to live in the moment, you are free to savor the many miracles that create life and sustain it.

15. **It is one thing to speak of the miracles that are inherent in life, but quite another to deal with the daily struggles of an aging body. How can we make sense of this struggle?**

Although this may be difficult to accept, it is simply a matter of perception. Much of the anguish that belongs to aging is the anticipation that today's problems are harbingers of tomorrow's more serious difficulties. Today's stiff leg may not work at all tomorrow. Yet, when a baby begins to walk, lacking the wit to know better, the toddler thinks it is funny to fall down. He thinks it funny when he staggers, and is not troubled by the endless repetitions required to learn to walk. You laugh as well because you know the child will grow stronger and more adept, and be more able. This developmental practice is viewed as charming or entertaining. By contrast, when difficulties are observed in the elderly, either by themselves or by others, it is viewed as a sign of negative things to come. But still there is much to be said for creating distance, observing from the outside, and trying to maintain some detachment in the face of these disquieting bodily changes.

16.   Can you describe the process of aging into awareness of spirit?

From the moment of birth, an individual begins to build the essence of what they perceive as self. Further details are added by lifelong experiences, family and society. The process of letting go that is a part of the end often takes away each of these layers, one at a time. The first layer that is given up may be the world of work. How many people you know define themselves by what they do, or did, who they were in their social circle, and who they were in the world of making money? But where does that money take them now? Through the years it has supported their family, and allowed them to define their worth as a successful, productive human being. The advantages have been of considerable importance, but beyond this, the role of worker often keeps people from truly knowing themselves. Who you are as a person has little to do with what you do. What you do to earn your living only relates to your livelihood. Who you are is where you actually reside in soul and spirit. And so the work falls away. In retirement, you hear people speak of the person they used to be, and usually each definition is external. As time goes on the end of life approaches and it becomes apparent that what counts most is the work of the soul's development. To the extent that people reflect on this, it is to the good, but more often than not, and particularly when still employed, the statement is, "This is my job. This is who I am." The true journey is to find the being, not the doing.

At the same time that work is dropped, physical changes may occur. The young believe their vigor, vitality, and looks will stay with them into the far distant future. It is hard to imagine, as they live each day, that what seems possible today will not be possible a year from now, as imperceptibly and implacably, the body shifts. Suddenly, one looks in the mirror and is dismayed to find that change has taken place. However, these physical changes are in many ways a beautiful, prolonged meditation on impermanence. It is just another opportunity to explore, reassess and live in the moment, but it is difficult not to feel these losses as little deaths. "Who am I, if I am not fit? Will there be continued love and value in my life?" The struggle with these questions is essential to your soul's development. For the person who is aging, and for those who love them, the task is to come to peace, recognizing the flame that burns within, and paying homage to the inner beauty that is God's gift to all.

17.   Aging progresses, infirmity becomes the fact of life. When the mind fails as well, what is left?

The most difficult losses an individual can sustain across time are memory and the ability to reason. You agonize and question, "Who am I if I cannot think, if I cannot reason as I did before? Where is my soul, if not in my mind?" Be assured that your soul resides in your beating heart. It is always available, regardless of any changes that occur. All changes are a valuable lesson offered in true lovingkindness, but still may be deeply resented. No longer able to fulfill the expectations that others had of you, you are now accepted for your soul's true value. You move from being loved and respected for what you can do, to being loved because you simply are. What remains is your value as one of God's beings.

18.   And dignity? In the face of all the losses of the body, how does one retain dignity?

Do not worry about your dignity, for dignity is of the spirit, not of the failing body. Individuals should not be embarrassed by changes in body which they cannot control. Normally, loss of control can be viewed as disgraceful and humiliating, but when health and body fail, it can become a part of daily life for many. However, their dignity does not rest in physical being, but in the nature of their souls. For all who rest in God's light there is dignity. They are pure souls and always able to move to the higher realms. On the more practical level, continue to treat an individual, no matter how frail and physically challenged, as an honored human being, fully worthy of this respect. When treated with dignity, dignity is maintained. If those around them treat the elderly as objects, or act as if they were children, or mock them, it is a painful and sad ending to their lives.

19.   The phrase often used to describe this stage of life is that the elderly are in "God's Waiting Room". In this instance, they wait for death. What is a better way to view this?

What a blessed opportunity, to live in God's Waiting Room, and yet all on earth are actually in God's Waiting Room, seeking their chance to enter that place where all is understood, and protection is universal. God's Waiting Room can be a place for deep reflection and an opportunity for grace, removed from cares, removed from obligation, finally given the freedom to become the spiritual being that on some level you have always yearned to be.

20.   Then God's Waiting Room can be viewed as a retreat and a cloister?

As families become busier and more fragmented, the elderly are being housed in institutions with increasing frequency. Though this housing may be very beneficial and benign, the tendency is to view them as places apart, a convenient solution to provide safely for those who are no longer productive or independent. In fact, they can be transcendentally beautiful cloisters, providing each individual with an opportunity for awareness and development of their higher level of being, while still enjoying this life. Still, one is not easily removed from the conditioning of a lifetime, and it is difficult to perceive matters in this way. Rather let all individuals see the beauty of the moment, the beauty of the opportunities that are presented to them and let them mourn no more, but seek God in those hallowed halls in which they walk, or totter, or perhaps are wheeled, in those days that precede the great awakening for each of them.

21.   How can we connect and relate with the elderly person evidencing unreasonable behavior or dementia?

For some, a sudden event such as a stroke, heart attack, or debilitating illness, brings them to a state of helplessness where much of who they were before is lost. For others, letting go is a more gradual process, where the awareness of loss dawns slowly. This can be a troubling and painful process. The greatest effort may be required when dealing with someone who is losing their ability to reason. As their ability to respond within societal bounds diminishes, they seem to demonstrate more and more of their worst qualities. At the same time, if you allow yourself to love that soul through this distressing disguise, through the tattered remains of what you used to see, you will come to a place with them which quite often is magical and well worth the wait. For some, and even more so for their families, it is not a long goodbye, but a long awakening, a long dawning of awareness after much pain and anguish and confusion and rage.

22.   What happens when memory fades and only the present moment exists?

When this happens the path is made easier in many ways, for it allows the individual to focus on the power of each moment. Even in dire circumstances there can be moments of great appreciation. To give an extreme example, a person in a hospital intensive care unit may not be allowed to drink because they cannot have fluids by mouth. They are permitted ice chips, and they will find bliss in the sense of a chip of ice on their parched lips. In that moment, they find heaven and peace, and perfect gratitude to those who brought them this gift. Similarly, as an individual struggles through a difficult morning, the fact that someone walks by, gently touches them on a shoulder, and says, "It is so good to see you.", is an opportunity to experience the full brilliance of God's grace in the act of another.

23.   What of the truly demented, and the advanced Alzheimer's patients. How do we communicate with them?

If we speak of communication as a product of logic and reason, dementia is a death sentence. But this is not so, for logic and reason do not rule all our communications. Communication at its best is heart to

heart and soul to soul, bound neither by words or the
habits of a long lifetime. Allow yourself to open to this
new dimension and enter into this place of grace with
your loved one. Although their ability to communicate
with you on your verbal terms diminishes, their capacity
for the soul to take flight remains undimmed and they
remain loving and caring individuals. It is their mind
and their body from which they are detaching, and the
soul leaves, pure and untainted, only when it has
learned what it needed to learn. And yet you wish to
communicate with your loved one, and this is a struggle,
for the tools you wish to employ are not the tools that
will be understood. The best avenues for
communication are not through words, or through the
use of the mind, but through touch and caress and
warmth and texture. Be available on that level, and the
message in your heart will be heard directly as it enters
their soul.

If you wish to show kindness to those who are
demented, offer small objects of softly textured
materials, perhaps woven, crocheted, or knit. As they
touch it and hold it, they are surrounded by your
prayers and loving thoughts. It brings them healing, and
brings you much good as well.

Together at Last

My father was a clever man. More clever by half than most of my friends' fathers who were good and prudent and wise, but limited by their mundane perceptions of the world. My father was a magician, a person who caused the room to brighten as he walked in, transforming everything and everyone into participants in his drama. Such a father is truly wonderful, but like a play, often best appreciated from a distance. Consequently, I grew up as an observer, not only of my father, but of the world. My experience was in the context of his drama and that of my mother. I thought this was everyone's life, and yet as I matured I found it was uniquely mine.

I learned that my world lay balanced between my father's exuberant self-confidence and my mother's dour concern for all the difficulties that might occur. I longed to be a part of the light that surrounded my father, but found more often that it was my mother's pragmatic sphere that enveloped me. And so I grew to adulthood just outside the wonder.

As an adult I realized that my father's charm and childlike enthusiasm kept him happy, but often at great distance from his family. I was aware that I hardly knew him.

Resigned to this I went about the business of
adulthood, raising my family and trying to craft a
role as daughter to my aging parents. Life had
been both kind and unkind to my mother and
father. Although healthy and financially secure
they lost many of those they loved to war, their
parents in the concentration camps of Europe,
their only son in the rice paddies of Vietnam.
They lived in each moment as they could, but
still used the present to replay their pasts. Fear,
recrimination and isolation alternated with
joyous engagement, good times and laughter.

My father retired when he was 64, shortly
after the sudden death of a very close friend,
more brother than acquaintance. My mother once
again found her choices and world shaped by the
decisions and thoughts of her intimate stranger,
my father. Over the years there was
accommodation, but never reconciliation to the
experience of this last stage. Throughout this
period I was a professor in a university
psychology department. I was very wise, just ask
the many who found my words helpful, but with
my parents, I was still the child working my way
through the thicket of emotions that had grown
during a lifetime of misunderstandings and
unresolved conflicts.

Both parents grew more frail, but in
addition my father developed the early signs of
dementia. Always self-reliant and suspicious of
others, he was unwilling to listen to suggestions,

nor accept help in the long decline into his
twilight. If my parents went to dinner with friends
my father would frequently descend into bitter
arguments, ending friendships that rested on years
of good will and camaraderie. My mother, clinging
to the clever man who had been, berated him for
his short-comings and felt they were purposeful,
directed towards creating unhappiness for her. The
graceful athlete had become a bent and shuffling
old man, disheveled and confused. It was a sad
and bitter time of increased isolation, regret and
attempts at change, while steadfastly, if not
stubbornly, refusing to see what might be done to
ease the suffering, if not the pain.

My mother was a good woman, but
unyielding. Her view of herself did not allow
failure, and to suggest that she could not care for
my father, or deal with his rages, confusion and
even incontinence, was unacceptable. In spite of
adequate means, my mother did not have help
with my father, and even when he needed a day
care program, she only sent him two days each
week. In turn, my father, confused by
surroundings that were too complicated for him
to comprehend, became belligerent and paranoid,
sometimes loving but often angry at what he
perceived as unreasonable constraints. Battles
raged over driving and were finally won by my
mother, but at great emotional cost to her. My
parents' marriage had been a traditional one and
my father still controlled finances, paying the
bills and making their decisions on a daily basis,

although such tasks were far beyond the abilities of someone who no longer could reliably find the bathroom, or even recognize his own home, let alone his wife and daughter.

One dreadful evening my mother had a stroke during one of their frequent arguments. I was living in another state at this time and the Sheriff's department notified me by phone from the hospital. I made arrangements to have my father looked after until I arrived and flew down to find my mother in a coma, and my father even more confused and disoriented than when I had seem him two weeks previously. Clearly he needed temporary placement at the very least, and possibly it was time to consider a residential facility for Alzheimer's patients. Through a combination of coaxing and tranquilizers, I brought him to a facility across the street from the hospital where my mother lay in intensive care. In the weeks that followed my mother rapidly improved, my father moved to a more appropriate facility, and the long term reality of the situation became clear to my mother. After three weeks in the hospital she was transferred to a rehabilitation facility. Already able to walk and move about, this respite was to build her strength so that she could return home. Within two days of a phone conversation with my father where he said he only wanted her to go home so that he could take care of her, she decided she would have none of this. My mother fell twice, and slipped into a final rapid decline ending in kidney failure. She didn't need to die, but she could no longer live. May she finally have the peace she needed.

My father was now alone, safe, but living in a twilight world few could enter or understand. I returned to live in Florida shortly thereafter and I was able to see my father frequently. Over the months and years a pattern developed, and this was the greatest gift I had ever received. Each week I would visit, a box of chocolates in hand along with whatever he might need in the way of clothes or extra care. In his dreamy state he found my mother, not dead as in reality, but one of the residents living with him in his new home. Fanny couldn't speak, but she still sang bits of old songs woven into the fabric of her life. And how she could love. There was none sweeter, a loving saint in tattered sweater and diapers. They would dance and he would feed her, communion of the highest order.

We all would sit and talk, hold hands and kiss, sharing chocolates and feeling the presence of our souls and the many we had loved and lost together. My father had always been a magician, but finally I could ride his magic carpet with him. He no longer could do math problems in his head, or even remember to close his trousers, but he could finally give love, unhampered by fear, or preoccupation with the outside world. People used to say how sad it was that my father was demented. I answered that it was a gift of God for him and for me, a chance to live with him and the other residents in an extraordinary world of grace and goodness, each moment pure and whole and fully present, the past gone, the future unanticipated.

One evening my father fell while dancing. A broken hip and a final stroke ended his journey in this body. I will treasure these final years forever. I finally knew and was loved truly by the man who was my father.

CHAPTER V

HOUSING

Although many issues may demand attention at this time, the practical necessities of life still have to be handled with immediacy for the elderly. The most basic issue is shelter. For the frail and the elderly, it is usually what level of shelter is required, what levels are available and what levels are affordable. After shelter, it is nutrition, and then the need to be safe during the day and throughout the night. These needs, and their specifics, shape and prioritize all decisions. For example, a parent capable of living independently may not need to move from their residence, while one who needs continuous monitoring, or who cannot prepare a meal, or who cannot take a prepared meal out of the refrigerator and warm it, is at another level. The management of each of these issues is affected in part by the individual's ability to bear the financial costs of care, and frequently, this becomes a significant problem where issues around the parent's planning, effectiveness and choices cannot help but surface.

Encouraging your parent to be open about financial affairs while they still control their choices may be futile, for it involves surrender of power when they feel weak and buffeted by the circumstances that surround them. Because of this resistance, it is possible you will have to bear silent witness to what you view as the ineptitude and poor choices of your parents. Painful as it may be, you are not in a position to change it, nor are you in a position to change the mind of a parent who stubbornly says, "I am not getting help in the house," or "I am not putting my partner in a nursing home." You can be with them and you can emotionally support them. You can even offer suggestions and guidance, but only your parent has the authority to make these choices.

24.   Putting finances aside for the moment, what housing is most suitable?

Always, the first consideration is the physical safety of your parent. Without the assurance of physical safety, you will live in fear and concern for your parent's frailty and vulnerability, and your parent may live with these fears as well.

In these changing circumstances, parents will live in many places. They will live in their own home, and they may even live in your home, while others will live in places specifically designed for those who cannot fully care for themselves. Each of these situations, although they vary widely in comfort and appearance, will require adjustment for all concerned. Even the best of solutions will require a period of time before you and your parent are comfortable.

The issues will be, "Can my parent stay in his home? Must my parent move to a facility that will take care of him? Should my parent live with me?" These are choices that may evolve across time and circumstance. Needs, desires and financial means change, and there are many components that will enter into these decisions. What is most important, is the intent and the desire of those who are making these decisions and this transition together.

It is obvious you will have to address the issue of finances at this time. While finances are important, remember that when living arrangements are made, it is not necessarily how much money is spent, but how much heart is delivered. When you look for a new home for your parent, first look to your heart and to theirs. Although many physical aspects are relevant to this decision, the choice must stem from the heart, and the heart's desires. Is there a desire for community? Is there a desire for comfort? Is there a desire for privacy, or is there a strong need to have many people around? All of these considerations will inform the decision that is made. When your parent can no longer live at home and perhaps must have help available continuously, the time has come to consider communal living arrangements. It is paramount that your parent's actual needs be met in this regard, not your desire to fill the needs as you perceive them. Your parent may have one set of desires and needs that can be met by a certain setting. You, however, out of the best of intentions, may wish or imagine that your parent has other needs or concerns. Although a certain elegance of setting and dress may appeal to you, it is more important that your parent be comfortable in the setting of their choice.

There will ensue a dance between the reality and fantasy of parent and child as this exploration progresses. The specifics of the setting, decor and amenities are not important. What is important is the emotional warmth felt as you move within the space. If you pull up and find the building inviting, if there is warmth and caring, you will recognize it. In spite of difficult conditions, is the staff able to engage with all the residents in a friendly manner? Is there light present in the place, not just the light of electrical illumination, but the light of laughter, the light of pleasure, and the light of joy and perhaps even the light of God? Is there a spirit of merriment as well as safety, can the smell of good food be noticed? Is this a place that will feel like home, or will it feel like one of the many waiting rooms that your parent encounters when they go to a doctor? All of these are important questions to ask regarding the heart of the place. Do the people who work there serve out of some level of satisfaction, or only out of obligation and bitterness? Food prepared in bitterness will have no flavor. Food prepared and served in compassion will fill the soul. Each of these factors will strongly affect how pleasantly or unpleasantly the setting is experienced.

The requirements described are not specific to a given price range or category. That is a completely different issue which each individual and family must decide for themselves. The care required will also determine choice, but regardless of the level of care required and the finances available, let it be a humane place, a loving and compassionate location in which your parent can be who they are. Try to minimize the shift from their former way of being in the world. Let it be a gentle continuation, in a more supportive atmosphere, of all they have cherished throughout their years.

25. Regarding the new housing, there may be possibilities of bringing furniture from home or using furniture provided. How should one decide?

Most important is that something be brought from their past into the present, something that connects your loved ones to their history. They are not dropping their past, but taking it with them into a new environment. This does not necessarily mean that they need to retain their marriage bedroom set. For some, the furnishings of their adulthood, and even their childhood, may have great power. There are individuals who have furniture crafted by their grandfather, or even great-grandfather, and it may be central to their definition of home. For them, it would be nice to have a piece with meaning. If, however, furnishings have changed as the abodes have changed, emotional connections are somewhat less distinct. In all cases, it would be wise if they carry something from their past, such as a set of candlesticks with family history, mementos, pictures, including as well something that bridges to the new, something that is fresh and selected specially for this place, because this is not the last sad end of life, but the beginning of a time of opportunity and exploration.

By the same token, there will be those who wish to take no reminders of their past with them. You may want to make some decisions for them in this regard, saving

and storing photographs and mementos against the day
when they may have a change of heart.

26.   Is there a way to close the former
home and minimize the pain of leaving?

If both the parent and the child participate, this can
be a time of real union, of reflection on the joys, the
vicissitudes and the triumphs of the many years that
have passed, and even grieving for the losses. If the
parent is widowed, part of the grieving is for the partner
that is already gone. At other times, it is grieving for the
abilities, or the skills, or the strength that used to be
present, or in some cases, for the neighborhood that
used to be safe. In fact, closing the house is an
opportunity to review and refine all of the many events
and aspects of the years that have preceded this move. It
is an opportunity to review the physical space and the
objects within, not because they are of great
importance, but because they allow you to touch old
memories and hold onto them.

It is often quite surprising to go through the home
of someone who has lived there a long time, and, in
spite of many rich memories, see how few of the objects
actually have material value. Physical objects provide an
anchor for the review of events. Even if they are ordinary,
such as the placemats used on the little kitchenette
table, they can be filled with memories, with love, with
conversations, with strife, with recollection, and with
history. The act of going through the home when the
parent is leaving, or has left, can be a time of reflection

and revisiting. It is a sacred time, and the home, for just that short period, becomes a sacred place. Do not underestimate the healing power of letting go of that space with respect and reverence.

27.   How do you help a parent realize their home is no longer safe or appropriate for them?

Regardless of increasing problems, most often your parent will not yield on housing until circumstances compel them to do so. It is almost as if they are loathe to say the words, "I just can't do it. I no longer have it in me to be the person I was." In spite of the fact that they will be less burdened by responsibilities, and that their mood, comfort, and even joy will improve, this acknowledgment is resisted. Nevertheless, it is reasonable to begin discussing alternatives with them. For many, there gradually will develop a process through which decisions and change will evolve. The first struggle may be, "You really need help in the house." As this is managed another problem will emerge. Perhaps stairs may become a problem, or the sheer size of the home, or cooking. Some parents will accept help and accommodate to these changes, but sadly, this is not always the case. Your parent may believe that to be valued they must be productive. Consequently, there is much defeat and anguish around the issue of what they can and cannot do. And you struggle as well, worried about your parent having adequate food, safe shelter, and being free from harm in their own home. If there is stubborn refusal to consider any alternative, sadly you can do nothing. Then it will be a crisis, another crisis in their own health or in the health of a spouse, that will create the necessity to evaluate the situation anew. In some ways your parent may desire a crisis so that they can be free from the burden of choice. At some point they will agree to this choice, just as long as they do not have to accept responsibility for it. If you have discussed these issues in the past with your parent and have information on what resources are available, then when a crisis strikes you will operate from an informed position, and can inform your parent as well.

> **28.   Please speak to the guilt of a child who must move the parent from a cherished home into an institutional setting. How can the child deal with the feeling of letting their parent down?**

Such guilt is painful and comes from the sadness that you are unable to fulfill the parent's desire to live out their life in their own home. Your parent may have said, "Please, never put me in a home. Never make me live and die among strangers like a dog." These words cut to the bone, leaving you torn and troubled.

As you struggle, you find yourself at war over conflicting desires to be responsible and loving, while wishing someone else could be responsible and loving in your place. All of these feelings are part of a complex mix that creates a guilt so large and so deep that you recoil from the problems and prefer to stand back from them. This luxury is impossible because it probably falls to you, the child to handle the details and even as you do so, you must deal with the bitter fruit of your own mixed emotions.

It may be of comfort to recognize guilt as yet another form of grieving, a way of examining and accepting changes that have occurred. Hopefully, this troubled period will be followed by new awareness as well as the strength and confidence to deal with the troubled attachments of memory and history, so that both you and your parent will come to a loving connection untainted by worry.

29.   What if the parent refuses to respond to your efforts, and is unwilling to participate in these important decisions?

It is important to remember that you and your parent arrive at this time and place carrying the history of your relationship with you. Each of you reacts according to your experience of that history. Regardless of the nature of this past, there is no way to take control when control is not yours to have. There is no way to eliminate problems and smooth the path for someone who insists on increasing or creating their difficulties. There is little you can do. You can observe silently, and you can comfort yourself by letting each rejection and complaint be a reminder for you to connect with someone else whom you love, and from the heart tell them how much they mean to you. It may not improve the relationship with your parent one wit, but your soul will grow hugely from the attention and affection you both offer and receive.

Resolve now to avoid this problem with your own children. Although you may not be able to avoid a state of high drama and disaster with your parent, now is the time to let each blocked avenue be a clarion call for you to open communication with your children. Trust in their love for you, just as they have always trusted in your love, and work for the future so that the mistakes of one generation are not carried into the next.

30.   Sometimes in closing their home parents have to be separated. What guidelines are there for such a decision?

This is a very tough situation. The emotional equivalent of your thinking is, "I am killing one and saving the other." This decision speaks to the powerful beliefs you have about the value of living in the family home as compared to living elsewhere, even though living elsewhere may be the wiser choice. The question is not so much how to make the practical decisions, because the practical decisions will rest on who needs skilled care, who needs care that might not readily be available in the home, and financial considerations. The real issue may be that there is a greater attachment to one parent than the other. While it is altogether natural to be closer to one parent than the other, it is difficult to deal with the feelings of guilt and confusion that arise around this common circumstance. Once again, listen to your heart and honor your feelings. The task before you is difficult enough without the added burden of guilt over these feelings.

31. How can the child assume the tasks of the parent without experiencing or creating resentment?

In a practical sense, it is wise to ask the parent if they have any needs or preferences. Often they will say. "I don't need anything." Need is relative and perhaps what your parent means is, "If you love me, you will know." or "Act for me, decide for me." If this is the case, you must struggle with your own decisions. Make these decisions knowing that you are doing the best you can and slow down. Rather than doing the shopping for your parent as part of a busy routine, set it aside as a meditation on service, on love, on connecting with your parent. If it is done in that mind and in that spirit, what is chosen will be of service, regardless of outcome. Let generosity reside within you as you carry out these tasks of love.

32. And how to deal with the parent who sends you back to return something repeatedly, letting you know that no matter how hard you try you cannot satisfy them?

This is but another enactment of a dynamic discussed earlier, "Where can I control when all control is gone?" If the situation becomes so impossible that there is no way for you to deal with it, as your pain and frustration and mount, it might be wise to step back from your efforts and let it be. As long as your parent has one garment to put on, they will not be naked. Most important is that you understand this process for what it is, a connection, in some ways a dance, and in some ways an echo of past dances. Do not accept or own the annoyance or sense of failure your parent may wish to impart, for it may only be their attempt to keep you closely involved with them. Relax and stay in the grace of your effort and your desire to provide love, if you can. If you cannot, then do the best you can.

33.   **Sometimes a wife has to place her husband where he will be safe and cared for, because she can no longer fulfill these functions. Is there a way to approach this kind of grief and guilt?**

For either the husband or wife faced with this problem there is guilt. It is easy to say there should be no guilt, but guilt abounds, for this good-bye is a complicated one. In all likelihood, the healthier spouse will remain in the home that has been their home together, surrounded by memories and recollections. In some ways, it will be hardest for them for they will feel the absence of their partner more than if they, too, had moved. Of course there will be pain due to failure of obligation. "I have failed the one obligation I had to my partner, which was to take care of them until death." This feeling resides deep in the heart, and is compelling even when the relationship has not seemed particularly pleasant or intimate when viewed by others. Nevertheless, the bond has been durable, and carried great meaning.

What may be most devastating is the change that is acknowledged when the partner says, "I am no longer a person who can take care of others. I no longer will take care of you. I no longer can." The spouse must deal with the failing partner's health, with their care, and even finding a place that is suitable for them. Next, they must deal with the sense of grief and loss and shame that is attendant to placing their spouse in an institution, no matter how pleasant. This is quite different from the guilt a child might feel, as the shame emerges from a personal sense of failure, a sense of not being adequate to meet the responsibilities of their marriage vows.

New Thresholds

As you take this first, most painful step in adjusting to the changed reality of you and your loved one, it is most important not to falter, to trust your love and good sense to find the best solution for your parent, spouse or loved one. For me, the task began with facing the fact that I had to take control and determine the future for both my Mother and Stepfather, happily married for 31 years. At 88, Mother was still doing fairly well taking care of the two of them. In spite of a bad case of shingles ten years previously that had left her in chronic pain from nerve damage, she still did all her own baking and cooking, played cards, and enjoyed a joke.

Though we did not know it at first, my Stepdad had been advancing into dementia (Alzheimer's, perhaps) over the course of eight years. Now at 93, his condition was deteriorating rapidly. At first we made the usual allowances for memory lapses, but denial became impossible. Even Mother acknowledged his condition, but his disposition remained sweet and amiable. He did not wander, and he continually expressed his love for Mom. She struggled as he became incontinent, as his actions became a threat to their safety, and he was no longer able to walk unassisted. Gradually, her health diminished. Her housekeeping deteriorated; she could not prepare meals; she did not smile. My husband and I, by plan, lived just twenty minutes from them, a good thing as the calls for help came with greater frequency, tinged with anger and bitterness at us, and at life. Finally, when my husband and I felt the situation was killing Mom and choking our lives, I made the decision to place my Stepfather in an assisted living facility.

When I sat down with Mother to lay out the facts, I had already done much research on facilities that would take residents in Saul's condition. I knew locations and prices, had visited places and interviewed staff, and had settled on one place, though I had an alternate available. Mother agreed readily, relieved that the decision was mine and not hers. She was bereft at living without him, at being unable to fulfill

her loving duty to care for him. At the same
time, she was frightened about economic
survival. They both had worked hard and earned
modestly. A lifetime of saving would be wiped
out by two years of nursing home fees. And how
was she to survive, she wondered. Our
reassurances could not lift her mood.

   I had thought things would ease up for all
of us once the enormous burden of caring for
Saul was taken out of Mom's hands. What I did
not expect was that Mother's condition would
take an immediate and drastic turn for the
worse when she no longer had him to care for.
She grew weaker and more helpless. We went
from doctor to doctor as she lost her appetite,
lost weight, withdrew, and became hostile. With
only occasional glimmers of the mother I knew
to remind me of who she was, I began to pull
back emotionally. It was not possible to limit
contact because she was too needy. I tried to take
her to live with me for a short respite, but she
was even unhappier than I was, and asked to be
taken home after a few days. It was only two
months after she placed Saul in a residential
facility that she had a stroke. Now that she was
sick she no longer has to make decisions about
her future. Fortunately, she recovered from the
stroke totally, and during the period of
rehabilitation was placed on an anti-depressant
drug that slowly let the person she had been
emerge once again.

During the period of her recovery, I went shopping again. This time for a communal living facility for my mother. I wanted a place where there would be people with mental faculties as sharp and intact as Mother's. The social worker at the rehabilitation facility worked with me to bring Mother to the frame of mind where she was willing to leave her apartment, at least on a trial basis. Within a short time she agreed, and once again, she seemed relieved that the decision was not in her hands. The choice of living facility for Mother turned out to be a good one. That, coupled with the anti-depressant, literally brought her back to life, and to a relationship with me that is loving and accepting, providing a contentment between us that was seldom present before.

Do not expect this settling in at the new home to occur painlessly or rapidly. The first months may be spent in fault-finding. This may be followed by a quieting, and reconciliation with the setting. Slowly, interest kindles in the activities offered, friendships are made, and the days become comfortably busy. The same food that was terrible in the beginning, now is tasty. Mother attributes a large part of her recovery to a setting where she knows she is safe and looked after. Nothing is demanded of her that she cannot fulfill. She is no longer frightened that she will be stricken and unable to summon help. Even if she is unable to pull the cord in her room that calls for assistance, someone will be in to check on her if she does not show up where expected. She also knows if she is ill and does not feel up to going to the dining room, food will be brought to her, and nurses and aides will look in on her.

Through the early days of this evolution, I often questioned myself. Was I railroading my Stepfather into an institution to make my life easier? Was I making decisions for my Mother in a loving frame of mind, or to get myself off the hook? I reminded myself frequently that I was a good and loving person. I accepted that I might make mistakes, but they would not be major if I acted from my heart. Together Mother and I have passed through confusion and pain, and now know peace.

Do no harm to others and love the angry for it is their cry for help. Heal with your touch and your words.

CHAPTER VI

WE'RE NOT GOING TO HURT EACH OTHER, ARE WE?

Regardless of the best intentions, all participants in this unfolding drama carry history and reactions from a lifetime of experiences. Parents may have found methods of communication that worked for them as a couple, though unpleasant to observe. Many couples thrive on bickering and sarcasm, however painful it seems to others. Now, however, they no longer can turn to each other while engaging in this verbal dance, and they seek other outlets. If these circumstances are familiar, your adaptation may have included infrequent contact, but now it is harder to avoid these distressing interactions, and you may even become the target. It is likely that you have experienced this previously, but now disengagement may not be possible. The real struggle here is that communication between you and your parent must continue, decisions have to be made, not at some future time, but in the present. Yet, when difficulties arise old patterns are reawakened, and even if there is no direct intention to cause pain, pain ensues.

34.   The parent retains the power to hurt the child. It may be the final source of power they possess. Is there a way to deal with the abuse of this power?

There are many ways to deal with this problem, though few ways to change it. To begin, remember you also retain the capacity to hurt your parent and these wounds within family are often the most fiercely inflicted and deeply felt. Some segment of family life is always about power, and when traditional power is gone there may be few domains in which your parent can exercise control. In spite of all this, when you are with your parent do not be distant or disengaged, even though this connection may require tremendous effort. Previously you may have disengaged rather than remain present, withdrawing to prevent unpleasantness. Now it is time to observe the process, being a witness to what occurs but still fully and directly offering love. Look for a new way to remain connected, for instance, it may be easier to share a piece of cake than to share a thought or feeling. This simple act may be less contaminated by old habits of judgment and criticism. Find that dimension in which sharing can happen unhindered and unfettered, and accept that occasionally distress will arise. Take the moments that are most peaceful as gifts and seek to treasure those, while dealing dispassionately with the more unpleasant aspects of creating new avenues of communication.

35.   **It is not simply a matter of ignoring repeated barbs and old complaints from the parent, but of handling the resulting pain. What can we do?**

Most people prefer to avoid confrontations, but each of you has the right to speak out when you are hurt by your parent's words. If it has been your habit to disengage and ignore, this is your chance to discover a more useful and ultimately satisfying avenue of response. Remember, although individuals have the power to cause pain, they also have the power at any moment to reverse a lifetime of pain and anguish by a loving touch, kind word, or smile that speaks to the soul. It is this possibility of change for the better that is most important. This is often forgotten in the rancor and dismay that surrounds these troubling times.

36.   **Children see themselves as parenting the parent. How can the paradox of this situation be handled?**

No matter what events may occur, it is critical to remember the child is never the parent. In contrast to earlier times you now may be the provider of care, or the person who performs the instrumental tasks of daily living, but there is no way the natural connection between you and your parent is modified. No matter what your feelings, the history of the relationship, your reluctance, or even your resentment at assuming this task, there may be nowhere else for your parent to turn.

This is a difficult time, even more complicated in this society which infantilizes the frail, and believes those who cannot care for themselves are somehow less than full human beings. You must recognize that the soul remains intact regardless of the assaults of age and infirmity. It makes no difference whether the individual's loss is of mind, physical stamina or status. These losses are disturbances of the vessel, not of the contents.

37.   Since both the parent and child have the power to hurt, what of the urge on the part of both to get even for past slights and hurts?

Sadly, this dynamic can continue, often until the very moment of death, denying both of you those simple phrases that would bring you peace. As much as there is the power to hurt, to recall and bring to the present past hurts, there is equally the opportunity to embark on an adventure and a connection that is different than any you have ever known together. It is not so much a question of letting the past fall away, but of being so much in the present that the past is distant and irrelevant. This is far easier said than done, but you must be sensitive to those moments in which you are fully connected and treasure them.

If your parent lives in your home, this entire process can be more difficult. You cannot adjust the amount of time you spend with your parent under these circumstances, and this may make getting along a constant trial. Yet each meeting is a fresh opportunity, for the moment is now. Even words spoken five minutes earlier are in the past. At first this concept may be difficult to act upon and much thought and even rehearsal may be required to develop a sense of presence in the moment. There may be hours of thought leading to a few moments of heartfelt conversation. As you practice with this new outlook it will become easier for you, and both you and your parent will begin to open to a newer, more intimate level of communication. There will be less preparation and far more pleasure, a world of discovery unfolding and awaiting you both.

As the flowers in the early spring are tender, so are your new feelings and behaviors. Protect and praise them.

CHAPTER VII

EMOTIONAL RESPONSES AND NEEDS OF CAREGIVER

Regardless of your best and most heartfelt efforts, your parent may not be able to change or see things differently. This is not unusual, but you may still experience this as a painful dead end. Hopes and fantasies of finally having a warm and intimate relationship with your parent fail to materialize and once again, you are forced to accept unwanted limits on this, your connection with your parent. No matter how much you want and need your parent's approval, respect and love, you fear it is not to be given.

38. How can the caregiver remain balanced in this situation?

To remain balanced is to attend to both your parents' needs and your needs in this time. Yet it can be difficult to offer an open heart to those who berate you. Remember that while their words have the power to harm, words are not truth just because they are spoken.

What is said may have little connection with fact, but rather they are the expressions of someone who is physically weakened, emotionally distraught, angry and beholden to you. An ongoing struggle over power and control will evolve as both of you define your new world. Although it is difficult to continue messages of love and compassion regardless of what is returned, still, consider this an opportunity to offer compassion without expectation of return, to make an offering of love from your heart. With so much pain and upheaval it is unwise to invest all your emotions in this relationship, so hold fast to aspects outside your relationship with your parent. Now is a good time for you to seek other paths to feel whole, beloved and comforted. Allow yourself to benefit from the support and caring of those around you, and give them the opportunity to surround you with the warmth and approval that is denied by your parent. Do not hesitate about imposing your problem on others, for in giving this gift of comfort to you, they provide for themselves as well. Nourishing you, they feed their own souls.

39.   We bear the secret shame of parental rejection. How can we find the courage to speak of this pain?

It is unfortunate when accusations by your parent feel shameful, as opposed to merely misdirected. Remember this sense of shame belongs to you and does not necessarily stem from the accusations. It may even come from old lessons you learned as a child. At the same time, the more fully you can be yourself and share what you view as undesirable qualities in yourself, the more fully you will know you are accepted for who you really are, not for the mask you show to the world. Be honest and comfortable in the awareness that this is who you are. Accept that there will be spots and blemishes, both in the perceptions of others, and more importantly, in your perception of yourself. The more open your heart is to others, the more you will receive, from them, from God and ultimately from yourself. The more willing you are to be fully yourself, the fewer problems you will have in absorbing and dealing with the many issues that arise in these times.

40.   This implies a loving respect for your own worth. How can this be nourished when so much attention must be focused on current difficulties?

It is true that much is required of you, but often it is this difficult work that you are doing that finally allows you to acknowledge you are worthy of the respect you desire. Caretaking must be offered, but to be caught in a reaction to the behaviors and unkind words of your parent allows you to be wounded in a way not intended, and even if intended, is intended by someone with diminished capacities of judgment.

In the midst of all this activity remember, if you do not care for yourself, it is unreasonable to expect anyone else to care for you. Driven as you are to use your resources to their very limits, and succeeding in managing a difficult and fluid situation, see yourself as the thoroughly capable individual you truly are. It is entirely appropriate to say, "I want to take care of me. I am a worthy creation of God. If God loves me and respects me, how can I not love and respect myself?"

Under some circumstances you are unable to do anything. You may be required to stand by as people you love choose to live out their lives in whatever manner they planned long ago. The most painful circumstances occur with those who have always expected to be miserable and unhappy, to die abandoned and forgotten. If this desire is strong enough, the most helpful ministrations on the part of family and friends will not alter the outcome. It is almost as if they are bent on fulfilling every one of their dire predictions. Then you might bear witness, available within your limits, and know the love you have is being offered as fully as you can offer it. Do not demand blind acceptance from yourself of all that your parent says or does, but rather, seek to connect at some level, regardless of the difficulty. It is arrogance to believe that you are all powerful and capable of altering anyone's life, or even alleviating their misery. The best you can do is offer your help and accept your personal limits, for it is their work to be done. Focus on the possibility to expand your own soul and your own heart.

In the midst of all these painful realizations, do not forget that the end of life need not be a lone journey, but can be shared. To be able to ease the dying of another is a gift, and those who participate benefit and gain understanding as they engage in this great journey. Death is the part of life for which all else is preparation, and the one transition in existence most essential to soul's growth. Privileged to share in this process, you not only grow personally, but gain through participation in the evolution of another.

Gone But Not Forgotten

It was finally over, Father gone, buried beneath the hard, dried earth of South Florida. The years of hoping for acceptance from him, anguish of rejection and a lifetime of sad childhood memories were ended. In the long months before his death she stayed by his side, encouraging him to eat, badgering the nurses so that he would receive better care, and always, throughout everything, always loving him. She hovered around him, hoping to see him smile, and waiting for him to tell her he loved her. She was 67 years old and she still wanted Daddy to say she was a good girl.

Somehow Margaret had thought that with her Father's death she could finally find some peace. At least she would have the comfort of knowing she had done all she could for him. Instead, her sadness came in waves. First she grieved for the loss of physical connection, then for being an orphan, losing the one person left who knew her as a child, and lastly she grieved for the loss of opportunity to finally hear her father say that he loved her.

And at the end, he slipped away, not perfect, but perfectly Daddy, the one she loved. She found life without him was not easy. Her routine for so long revolved around him and her desire for his recognition and approval, and now all she had was time, time to think and time to heal. With time's passing, her strength and confidence return. There will ever be a place in her heart for him and for the memories of loving him. In the spring she will plant a garden. Daddy always liked flowers.

CHAPTER VIII

REGRETS AND GUILT

Time makes its inroads, circumstances change again and again. One day you may find yourself with a parent who says: "What have you done with my money?" or in a pleading voice begs, "Why can't I live in your house? Take away my pain. Why aren't you here today? I'm weak, help me." These utterances and the neediness they convey may be totally out of character, and still you are left bewildered and beleaguered, searching for the independent parent of the past now present only in your memory.

41. What happens to people whose personalities change radically as they age?

Children do not want their parents to diminish, but to remain vigorous, and most important, familiar. In spite of these wishes, unfamiliar qualities and even unpleasant characteristics begin to emerge. As the veneer of accepted behavior wears away you wonder, "Where within this new set of behaviors and reactions does my parent exist?" You and your parent now enter a most difficult stage, not because you cannot feel their pain, but because much of what they say is distressing, painful and almost intended to drive you away even as you wish to help. While this may be experienced as mean and hurtful, it is merely another phase in the long process of letting go. Do not make much of this troublesome passage. Later it will be easier in many ways to connect with the parent who is past this rage and confusion, no longer driven by nameless fears even though their grasp of events and recall may be diminished. And yet it is in these difficult early times that work needs to be done between you with your full memory of your parent as a vibrant person, and the parent who now seems just a shell of their former being. It is not this shell to whom you must relate, but to the person within. This requires significant awareness and objectivity on your part, for it is always hurtful to be accused or found wanting.

While many responses are possible at this time, hold fast to the bond of your history. Often it is helpful to look back to a time of vital and satisfying connection between you and your parent, recall the emotions of that moment and bring them forward into the present. If, however, the past was always troubled and painful, and those memories are a trial to recall, you are left to reach out solely as an act of loving service, hoping your parent arrives at an oasis of greater receptivity. Have patience, for even if this receptivity is never achieved, it is good to stay in the moment. Accept your personal disappointment so that untainted by bitterness you may move forward.

**42.   It is hard to leave the desires and
demands of the parent unfulfilled.
How can reasonable expectations
be established?**

Limits are based on an evaluation of your parent's
needs and your ability to fulfill these needs across time.
These limits must be within the bounds of your
tolerance, and within what is necessary for your
survival, even more so than the survival of your parent.
As hard as this is, if you do not set these limits, you will
reach a point of saturation and will no longer be able to
accept demands of any nature. Guilt, resentment,
anguish and all the game playing that creates negative
feelings and strain within families need to be
minimized. You may not be able to stop your momentary
reactions of guilt and shame, but you can stop yourself
from integrating them and making these feelings part of
your being. Be aware when this is happening to you, and
do not force yourself to do that which has become so
painful. Regroup, assess your needs and take care of
yourself with compassion and understanding. Taking
care of yourself now will allow you to continue to take
care of others later.

Letting Go of the Pain

Let yourself find a quiet moment. Settle
into an inviting place, a comfortable chair or
pillow on the floor. Soften the lighting in the room
and surround yourself with comforting scents,
incense or candles, warm and inviting. Allow
yourself to feel nourished and supported.

Lightly close your eyes and breath slowly
and evenly. At first this will feel forced. Relax into
the process, and as you settle, focus on your
breath as it moves in and out of your chest.
Visualize your breath coming in and surrounding
your heart, warming it and bringing comfort.
Continue to breathe, imagining that you are
breathing in and out of your heart. As you
continue, allow the pain and sadness that you
have stored in your heart to surface, see it and
breathe it out. Be aware that the pain has been
real, but you do not need to carry it in your heart
always. Let the breath release your pain, and as
you exhale, let it leave your heart. Continue as
peace settles in around you, releasing the pain
into the quiet. Go forward with God's love.

CHAPTER IX

SPIRITUAL WORKSHOP

It is human nature to hold onto all that is familiar, but not all parents are blind to the negative aspects of their changing circumstances. As their world grows smaller now that friends and even family are gone, they will know increasing loneliness. Both you and your parent may feel this isolation and desire change, but the means for change may not be clear to either of you. Beset by losses and the intense emotions they provoke, your parent may become immobilized, and you struggle to help them find their way.

**43.   Sometimes the parent becomes
         depressed and despairing as relatives
         and friends die, and they live on alone.
         What can be done to help them?**

This is a painful experience and yet an opportunity for soul's growth. For many the problem is that strangers cannot replace lost loved ones. "Strangers. How can I laugh with strangers, and take pleasure in their company. Only my family, my good, old friends and people who share my history and my memories can make my heart smile." In some ways, it even feels disloyal to allow pleasure into the heart when so many have died. "How can I be happy when everyone I ever cared about has died? How can I, the sole survivor, let myself find pleasure?" This profound sadness and pervasive sense of loss must be transformed before your parent begins to reach out to you and to others. Further, in addition to being depressed and isolated, your parent may be suffering from physical complications. Malnutrition and poor self-care can come from the same sadness that numbs every day of their lives. These changes may be so gradual that they are hard to detect. Once you recognize the problem it is wise to seek every means available to reduce it. This can include group meetings to discuss issues and provide support, while social service agencies may be able to provide additional caring and nurturing. You may find that medical intervention is necessary as well. Although we speak of soul's work and spirit's work, there is much to be said for facilitating this work with the wonders of modern chemistry. Remember, do not underestimate the power of a loving visit, perhaps with food offered, and with compassion. You should not despair, for the opportunity is always present for your parent to move into a lighter time.

44.   For the elderly, loneliness is everywhere. Please help us to understand what can be done.

Loneliness is a corruption of the capacity to be alone in reflection. Comprised of the fear of being abandoned, left out of life's flow, it is the consequence of a multitude of wounds across time and a lifetime sense of failed expectation. There is a focusing on the unpleasantness of each change which contributes to this feeling of loneliness. Preoccupied by the accumulated weight of losses and changes, there arises an inability to look outside themselves and their pain to all the things that used to provide distraction and pleasure. If only they can reach out to make a loving connection, with each other, a pet or even in awareness of nature, this isolation can be undone in a moment. You can help them to be aware of the faintest lifting of the darkness and to appreciate it, for even the smallest light in a dark room is sufficient to show the way, and if they cannot or do not wish to see possibilities, at least you know you tried.

Loneliness does not arise out of lack of company or lack of opportunity, but rather can spring from a belief that the person who experiences this loneliness is not worthy, and they fear they will always be separate and outcast from others. This does not necessarily come from being old, sick or frail, but stems from the belief that they lack some essential quality and can no longer hide this flaw from others. They believe the mask behind which they have hidden for a lifetime has fallen away and they stand exposed. For them and for you as well, it is important to squarely face this fear. Help your parent to see themselves in all their richness, and see the same thing as you look into your own heart and mind. If you are able to feel that God's love is present, accept this and there is no need for anyone to live in loneliness. If not, the heart can still be open to allow the pain of old wounds to fall away.

45. How can the soul develop when all of life is intent on the here and now?

Living in the material world does not automatically prevent spiritual awareness and development. The soul can expand at the realization of the beauty of a drop of dew on a blade of grass, just as the heart catches at a baby's smile, and sometimes you are gifted with an incredible sense of peace and awareness. Even in this secular society it is possible to do spiritual work. Look back to those times when you had a special awareness, a grace note, a moment of everything coming together despite the harried quality of your life and you will see that development blossomed. Often it is the pause within the fray that has the greatest meaning. Develop and savor the ability to put down the task of the moment, take a deep breath, and send a kind thought to someone you love, even yourself. This is soul's work.

46. What is the place of prayer in our lives?

The greatest gift in difficult times is the power of prayer. Prayer can evoke peace, comfort, and entry into God's light, for God enters at the slightest call and request, bringing compassionate peace to all who ask. For someone who says, "I have not prayed before; it is unseemly that I do so now," let them be assured that God is willing to enter the heart of all who wish God to be present.

This prayer might be said by those seeking
peace and comfort.

Hear my pleas as I call to you in this difficult hour.

I am afraid and feel weak, fearful that I will not
master the task at hand.

Please give me courage so that I may rest in
the light of your love.

47.   How do we come to terms with our own mortality?

In spite of their stated belief that the soul might live on, for most in the Western culture, death is seen not as a transition, but as an end. If this end is viewed as a disappearance into nothingness rather than a flow from beginning to end to beginning, then there is fear for all is lost. It is the understanding of this fear that will enable you to come to terms with the mortality of your body. Allow yourself to believe that death is an opportunity to shed life's care and pain, and all the struggles of your years. Yet it is not simply a physical release, but a time of healing for the soul. To move from fear to an awareness of the full circle that contains both life and death is your life's work.

48.   How can one change awareness while hampered by regrets?

Some people face death without regrets. That is not

to say that nothing happened in their past that is worth regretting, or that they are unaware of what is left undone or unsaid. It is rather the recognition that these events are in the past, and no longer have impact or reality in the present. Regrets and guilt on the part of your parent as death approaches are distractions that prevent awareness of all that is present in the moment, the connections that are possible, and the transformation as the body ceases and the soul emerges free of the form that no longer serves it. Regrets and guilt on your part are like static, interfering with the attention and focus necessary to attend to your parent's passage. If there are words that need to be said to bring you both comfort, say them. Usually, a quiet touch, a hand firmly held, will say even more. There is neither need nor value in dwelling on regrets at this point in time. That stage is passed. The only function regret has is to teach you forgiveness of your own failings, and to change behavior you now see as unproductive, hurtful or wasteful of the moments available in a lifetime.

49.   What is the true function of mourning?

Mourning has been present in the human condition since prehistoric time, and an important aspect of man's development. In many ways, all life is a process of mourning , for with each gain there is a loss, and with each change a good-bye. Until now we have spoken primarily of mourning the loss of vitality and promise. You mourn as well the transformation of the adorable infant into a troublesome adolescent, those who have touched your life and moved on. You mourn love denied, and opportunity lost. Each of these events is preparation for other losses, and eventually the final mourning of life

itself. If you become adept at mourning you become
adept at life.

50.   How does this help the person who is
burdened with deep sadness and anger
at life's condition?

When gold is refined, it goes through a purification
process, and the impurities rise to the surface to be
taken away leaving pure substance. So it is with the end
of life. Life is a refining process in which negative
qualities become apparent and can be burned away. The
anger and negative emotions that rise to the surface are
remnants of ego, and the only way to deal with these is
to let them surface and thus dissipate. This is painful to
experience, as is the sadness that often emerges at this
time, but all are part of the journey.

51.   How does the belief in punishment
and atonement relate to the
emotions of this time?

Punishment or atonement, both are sides of the
same coin, equally valid as constructions of minds
seeking to soothe fears, deal with regrets and as devices
to manage the unexplainable and unknowable. Each
person, as they pass from this life into the other, creates
the heaven, the hell or the purgatory of their expectation,
just as they created their perception of reality in this
lifetime. They will shape what they experience to reflect
what they expect to experience, and even the full

heavenly host cannot convince a person expecting hell to see anything but hell. All are offered compassion and love, but your parent determines what is made of this gift and where personal awareness will carry them. To add the fear of punishment to the fear of death is too heavy a burden.

52.   How is one to grasp this concept of the unknowable?

Start by asking whether this knowledge would change the way you live. All the stages of life would remain the same and one does not need understanding to benefit, to experience or to be blessed. For millions of years animals, including man, have been on this earth and only recently has the concept of gravity been explained. This does not mean that gravity did not exist. It simply means man lacked the knowledge and the vocabulary to explain what he experienced, but this did not prevent him from benefiting from the effects of gravity. So it is with the unknowable, undefinable universal consciousness. You do not need to fully comprehend or define it to live within it. Nor do you need to consistently understand and practice full awareness in each moment to be able to evolve and move forward. Just walk the path, confident it continues beyond the limits of your vision.

53.   How can people approach the end of life without excessive grief and mourning?

It is wise to recognize that grief and mourning are natural to life, especially during the later years. For all your life you have known that unpleasant changes awaited you, mostly as losses. So now you are faced with the reality of your own losses, not just because it is more of a struggle to get through each day, but for all your lost hopes and unfulfilled expectations as well.

Grieving is hard work that can become impossible if carried to excess. It becomes excessive when you can think of nothing but your losses, and despair colors your every action and response. To work through it, begin by honoring your grief, recognizing those components that are quite real and those you have borrowed from tomorrow. Then gather into your heart the attention, comfort and compassion offered from those you love, and from those who love you. Value it, even though you may be inclined to disparage it as pity. Do not forget the comfort that also is yours from God, and lastly, look for comfort in the arms of your remembered self from your past.

54.   In the arms of your remembered self?

Yes. Time and space are structures that are far more artificial than real. Although events occur sequentially in your world, it is always possible to bring past memories into the present. As your parent rests in their frailty, pain, or sense of aloneness at this moment, let them recall a time when they were at their strongest and most compassionate. Now bring that aspect and that remembered self to the fore. Let them imagine that person as a good friend offering support in this difficult time. This part of each of you is always available, regardless of how the body may fail. Just as the child within you is never very far away, so the strong, powerful, confident person within you is never far away, ready to be called forth to nurture, care for and protect when fears grow. At this point, it might not be possible to see any benefit arising from this exercise, but lacking vision have faith that God provides a safe haven.

55.   Is there a way we can bring gladness to our hearts?

Gladness is already there. It rests in the heart, but can be veiled easily by sorrow and doubt. While all wish for peace and gladness, this is not sufficient, for it takes a more conscious effort to overcome the pain that is harbored in the heart. You will find that happiness can lie in the smallest gift of life, if you are open and aware, so focus on small miracles, be it a kitten, a goldfish, or even a flower. Have living things with you always, surround yourself with the colors of spring and wear them. Remember that even in the autumn of life there are opportunities to grow. Do not allow yourself to become transfixed by the specter of a negative future, but continually be open to the wonder that surrounds you. Through prayer and awareness, positive thoughts will appear and energy enter. Arrange to have within your home objects, images and pictures that are meaningful to you. Reflect on these and seek the encouragement, happy memories, and even the light they may offer you. Do not be afraid to sit in reverie, for you will find there is much peace to be had, and that strength and lightness will enter.

A Hug in Passing

Take a moment now to be especially kind to yourself. Sit comfortably, breathe deeply and evenly while relaxing your shoulders. Now look back to the question and answer that touched you most. Read it once again, this time aloud.

Then let your eyes close, and allow the spirit of the words to fill you. Continue to breathe softly and deeply. Soften into the experience and the emotions of the moment. Feel that support and guidance which is always available to you. Though you may feel you are walking or running alone, know you are not unsupported in your journey.

The sands of time run out, through the glass they move from one dimension to another even as your own thoughts slide about. Let each moment, like each grain of sand be appreciated, observed, treasured and wisely spent.

CHAPTER X

FACING DEATH AND DYING

Even as all are born, so it is true that all will die.
Whether this death is viewed as a final end or as a
transition, it is required that you move from the known
to the unknown. If death as finality is the accepted
viewpoint, it is intensely feared because all would be lost
at the end of life. If death is viewed as transition from the
body and soul to soul alone, there is still much fear
surrounding it. This shift from the physical plane has
been generally ignored in this culture, and consequently
it is hard to imagine a world where you do not exist in
physical form.

56.   **How can we approach the end of life**
        without being overwhelmed by the
        fear of dying?

The shift from clinging to the body towards giving it
up occurs as far more effort is required to stay in body
than to leave it. It is a decision reached by each person in

their own way and time, for it is difficult to overcome the fear of dying while still immersed in the fear of living. If you are receptive to the continuation of the soul after death, the shift may be easier, but anxiety and apprehension are the usual companions of man in this work.

Anxiety may be relieved in many ways. Always the support of those you love and trust is welcome, as is warmth and tenderness, physical comfort, and familiar scents and sounds. The scents and sounds of nature, like the lulling sound of flowing water, as well as a soft blanket, all have the power to give comfort. The person is engaged in a long good-bye to all that is familiar, as well as to the physical self. Let there be someone to hold a hand or touch a shoulder, for very few are afraid of the dark when they are not alone.

Just as each person has their own way of dealing with life, they approach death differently. Some individuals will panic and some will be serene, and so it is for the observer. This is not a time for you, the observer, to react to each changing concern and condition with alarm, for the dying process involves many physical changes, and these changes themselves create an additional cascade of changes. At other times, these circumstances might propel action, but not now. For many, this is a time in which they work towards grace and a serenity they may not have known before. Just sit in witness offering support and comfort. Beyond that, nothing is required.

57.   Nothing may be required, but what can the child offer at this time?

As your parent seeks to move inward and face the very door to death, the world may offer a crescendo of distractions that take them away from meaningful focus. There may be a cacophony of demands and expectations of medical interventions, when the greater need is to focus on letting go. Caught in arguments, delays, doubts, questions, and the endless minutiae of distractions, it is difficult to settle in clear awareness. In many ways it would be easier to die in a space not so devoted to keeping your parent from dying, such as is found in hospice. There the silence, the peaceful quality of supportive, compassionate non-intervention allows the individual at the very end stages the space they need to make the transfer. There you can offer your parent quiet reassurance instead of frantic activity, and loving permission to quit this world.

58.   By transfer, you are referring to death?

Death has as many meanings as people have faces. In a society that does not generally believe in the endurance of the soul, death may be seen as the entrance into the great emptiness. For an individual who holds steadfast to such a belief, you can offer gentle comfort and support in the difficult passage through the last, perhaps painful, moments of their life.

For individuals who are open to the possibility of something beyond this life, there are two avenues they may take. One is that they are reassured by the awareness, knowing they will have the opportunity to continue beyond this existence. The other possible outcome, more distressing to them, is that since there is existence beyond this life, there will be consequences for what they did and did not do. They will no longer be able to hide from themselves, their choices, or their behaviors and their judgment is at hand. It is perhaps most painful for these individuals.

If you believe there is nothing beyond life, you may cling to this world as long as possible, grasp as much as possible, and assume all disappears in the moment of the last breath. If, however, you believe that there is life beyond this life, and yet you fear you will be judged and held accountable, you hold onto life filled with fearful anticipation and guilt, and each difficulty in survival brings you closer to the precipice of judgment.

59.   Please tell us more about this fear of punishment.

In life, many people feel they are monitored, criticized, and judged for their actions. Some people who believe the soul exists beyond this lifetime fear that punishment will be the consequence of their prior failures and poor choices. These individuals often struggle very hard to delay the end of their life because they are so terrified of what will happen to them beyond the moment of their death. This fear is an extension of fear they have carried before, and an extension of negative judgments that have been offered to them, or imposed upon them. No, it is not God's wish to punish, but rather encourage, support, and instruct. Abuse, even when given for ostensibly the best of reasons, is abuse. Love and compassion eventually will bring all to the light.

60.   What about medications, narcotics, antidepressant drugs to help during this period?

Each person will create the environment needed for their passage, and there is nothing intrinsically right or wrong with medication. There is no glory in suffering and there is no glory in pain. It is best to alleviate pain while maintaining consciousness, so that the individual does not slumber out of their body. Still, for some individuals, slumber can be the greatest blessing as their life ends. Be sensitive and responsive to the needs of each person.

61.   Sometimes it falls to the child or spouse to make a decision whether life support or heroic measures should be used to keep someone alive. What should be done?

Your parent or spouse may have wishes you are not comfortable meeting, and so there is great temptation to substitute your judgment for theirs. This should not be done, for it is wise at all times to respect the decisions of the dying in this matter. If they say, "When this happens, my time is over," then their wishes should be respected, regardless of your desire for a different outcome.

This decision is even more difficult when it must be made in the absence of any information about your loved one's desires. Here a reasoned decision is confounded by your own hopes and fears, guilt and fantasy and it is unlikely that anyone can be fully honest with themselves in these difficult times. The wisest and most compassionate way of approaching this question may be: "If I can let myself rest in the state where I truly love my parent and wish for them what is the very best for them, what are the options? Should they be on life support? Artificially fed? Should there even be any further effort to treat, or do I instead support them as they let go of life?"

Rarely when you stand in this light of compassionate love, will you make the decision to use extensive or invasive treatment to prolong a life that is ending. It is the caregiver filled with mixed feelings, upset at possibly being perceived as not caring, who decides to extend life further and further, even into anguish. This is a time when all should be encouraged to say their good-byes. Far better now than at the moment of death, for if graced with sufficient time, this is an opportunity to enjoy and acknowledge connection. Then, when the time shifts and it is necessary to let go, there will be no panic.

Meditation

Difficult times invite healing thoughts. Let this meditation support you in these final hours.

May God always go with you in your darkest hours.

May you experience the healing you so richly deserve, and the light with which all are surrounded as they die.

Breathe deeply into your heart and feel the light of God that surrounds you and brings you grace.

Let go of the need to see and allow the reality of experience to enter. Release your soul from the trap of your mind and live in your heart.

CHAPTER XI

CONSCIOUSNESS

Pain and suffering are not necessarily part of God's plan for man's spiritual development, but they are one of a set of possibilities. In fact, much of what troubles people now is unique to this time, when so many causes of disease and death have been eliminated. Only in the very recent past have large numbers of people attained great age, and thereby the opportunity and leisure to find meaning in the process of aging. In more ancient times, the learning opportunities were often those offered by the bitterest survival. Today, however, man may live to great age, but it is not automatic that man lives to great wisdom. Great age gives people the opportunity to spend many years examining their reality, their fate, and their illusions. Unfortunately, they may also have spent many years living in a manner that makes it uncomfortable for them to examine these very same processes and aging then becomes a great challenge.

62. **It is difficult to seek wisdom when pain and suffering are present. Under such circumstances what can one learn?**

When the body begins to fail, or pain prevents awareness, it is not time to escape, but to embrace the experience of the moment. A limb that does not let you stand, forces you to do something else. Often what it forces you to do is sit in awareness and quiet. There are many ways to deal with the suggestion the body is offering at this time. Some of you may choose to rush about, to seek any distraction in an effort to delay awareness of your changing reality. If you have not been attentive enough to self and soul, perhaps slowing down would be wise. Allow your soul to join in the process of settling into the moment. It is often said that attending to pain increases your awareness of it, but an equally valid statement might be that not listening to what is being said by your body or your soul will merely increase the likelihood of its repeating itself. This is not to say that bodies do not take on attributes and qualities independent of soul's growth, for the body is both a spiritual and mechanical thing, a complicated miracle of development, subject to difficulties and frequent surprises. What you as an individual pilgrim do with these surprises will make a difference in what you learn from them.

63. **Please clarify the difference between pain and suffering.**

Pain can be a clarion call to action, or the desire of some aspect of your self to be noticed and addressed, or even a state of being. It is in the moment, a present event.

Suffering is a somewhat different issue, a prototype for anguish, a reflex from past experiences. It has a more complex set of roots, and physical pain is but one cause of suffering. Suffering comes out of history and moves into the future as an emotional response to the physical experience. Suffering carries past memories of hurt, indignity and anxiety, and becomes anguish when it is anticipated that the pain will continue on and eventually invade all aspects of life. If allowed, suffering fills all space and time, expanding to the highest levels of fear, and the lowest depths of despair. It is a separate thing from pain, but a close companion and the issue is not what it is, but how to deal with it. It is best to separate the two, to remind oneself that pain is in this moment. If there is action that can be taken to diminish pain, then by all means pursue it. There is no virtue in the experience of pain for pain's sake. It is unfortunate that as individuals age there is pain that cannot be removed, an awareness and level of discomfort that will continue at all times. The task then becomes one of how to deal with this pain without the complication of suffering. Be in each breath, in each moment, respect the sensation, and then put it aside. The process of letting go of pain and transcending it allows the soul to grow.

64.   Why are we placed in body?

Although it would be easy to be glib, there is no absolute why to being in body. Physical form exists in the field of physical reality and that is where you are. Your body is as effective and trouble-free as any living thing could be in the physical world. In spite of that, across time it will fail, partially because it is subject to much abuse.

There are many pieces of machinery in homes and factories, and few are as tolerant or forgiving of the abuses that are heaped upon them as the human body is of those abuses it experiences across time. So it is not so much why does physical form have problems, but thank God for all its magnificence and the fact that it works as beautifully as it does. The soul is placed in this wonderfully complex physical form to see through the windows of the eyes and to use the power of reason present in the brain. That is reason enough to be in body.

65. Could we not do the work better as spirit?

Physical development unfolds along fairly predictable lines, and changes that occur with each age can be predicted. With spirituality, there does not seem to be a developmental model, and yet spiritual growth is the major reason for life's experience.

There is work that can be done as spirit alone, but the physical plane is needed to ground the soul, so that even the smallest step can become one of awareness. In spirit it would be far easier to just slip away from that which you do not wish to do, or do not wish to see. In body, you are compelled twenty-four hours a day to have awareness of your presence, and how much you allow yourself to settle into that awareness will affect how much you grow as an individual. After all, without body you would not have the discipline of removing yourself from the distraction of the flesh.

Given the values of today's society, much of the aging process requires letting go of the many vanities that make up the flesh and ego. Today life is shaped by intellect and ego as much as it used to be by the status of the family. Once aging removes some of the power of ego, there is opportunity to consciously move away from the habits of a lifetime releasing the many masks of role and status, gaining knowledge and wisdom in the process.

66.   Ego relates to doing. Does it relate to a spiritual life as well?

In many ways, doing has become increasingly powerful in this world. Most of your life is spent in a doing state. In simpler, less affluent societies, the doing provides sustenance and housing. In this society, blessed by plenty, the doing has expanded to a fulltime occupation, if not of work, then of pleasure. There is always a doing to be done. If it is not the job, it is entertainment or sports, not to mention television and shopping. All this serves as an endless seduction from stillness, yet only in the stillness of a moment of reflection can the full orchestra of the heaven be heard. In just a moment's pause, one can touch the heavens and be touched in return.

There is nothing intrinsically wrong with doing, rather it is that human existence depends on learning the balance between doing and being. A conscious gratitude for simplicity will serve you well in this regard, and you are then free to be fully who you are, naked of illusion, standing in God's glory.

67.   How do reason and thought relate to a spiritual life?

Reason does not shape the goodness of mankind. The fusion of emotion, intuition and love brings you to your highest self, and it is there that the soul resides. However, reason is not without function for it serves both body and soul. Thought is the vehicle of reason which allows one to solve problems, yet thought is not an end of and by itself. The connection of being and soul is made through heart and feeling, not through thought. The best and highest place is in heartfelt awareness.

On Being

We speak of doing and being, yet how do we develop the awareness of their differences. Doing is that aspect which can be calculated, summed at the end of the day, weighed for its value, crossed off on a list. Being, on the other hand, is as fleeting as a single beat of the heart, as light and ephemeral as a particle of dust floating through the air.

The goal of life in the world is not to eliminate doing, but to create some time and space in each day for awareness, being in each moment as you slowly watch it drift through

---

consciousness, awareness without direction or intent, but simple acknowledgment of all that passes through life. The following meditation might prove helpful in this endeavor.

Seat yourself comfortably erect, but not stiff. Allow your eyes to gently close and bring your attention to your breathing. Let your breath travel throughout your body, each breath bringing calmness and ease. Continue to breathe and allow your heart and mind to open. Allow space for everything, all thoughts, feelings and sensations. Notice all that comes to your attention and let it move on.

Reflect on your connection to the earth, as you sit and note all that surrounds you and is within you as well. The seasons of life change, fortune rising and falling. All that comes will pass away. Rest with a heart of compassion amidst all this change. Continue to sit in this centered awareness and when you are ready, open your eyes and move slowly back into your routine. Seek to hold this view of being so that you are totally present in all that occurs.

Do not let the questions of the past impede your future, but accept the doubts as gifts on the path to understanding.

CHAPTER XII

FAITH

Amidst the profound physical losses at the end of life, there is difficulty in accepting that spirit continues on, for if it cannot be experienced in body, how can it exist?

For those who believe in the existence of soul beyond death, little is needed other than knowing that they will have access on some level to those who have gone before, as well as to those who remain. However, it is difficult to convince individuals who believe only in the material that more awaits them beyond earth. Convincing them is not as important as supporting and comforting them in the moments of their passage. You cannot compel them to accept a belief that is foreign to them, and it may be sufficient comfort for them to rest in the arms of man as they draw their last breath. Those who believe in existence beyond life know that as they leave, they rest in the arms of God. Both paths provide comfort, and once the passage has been completed, all will see the reality beyond death.

68.   What do we say to those who believe God is simply wishful thinking?

Many believe that God is just a product of anxious and inadequate minds, created to put to rest fears that otherwise could not be managed. There is no way to convince the unconvinced, nor is it your obligation to inform, educate or convert others to your belief. It is not easy to influence the will of others. Individuals who wish to believe will do so, and individuals who feel compelled to deny may unfortunately do so as well. They have the opportunity to move beyond their doubts, or to stay within their limitations in this lifetime. Offer them a grander vision, and if they choose to accept it that is for the good, for it is an avenue to their own peace and comfort. If they cannot believe in God's love, they will follow their own path.

69.   Are there other paths to solace?

Many turn to other cultures to achieve peace. In some cultures, dropping the body is viewed as a positive transition, but in this society, although religious teachings support the enduring soul, people often live as though physical reality is all there is and only endings are seen. What ultimately will bring peace is an understanding that existence is possible beyond the body. Of course continuity of spirit rests in the memory of others, as well as on other planes. For those who do not have the faith that other planes exist, it is difficult to change their beliefs. No one needs an evangelist at death's door. Already distressed and worn, perhaps suffering and in pain, they may be unwilling to open to the spiritual at this time. Remember, each person, as they approach the end of their life, should have the opportunity to find the answers that are appropriate for them. Provide them with a loving environment, filled with compassion and your own belief about continuity, creating a space where they can feel comfortable. The knowledge of the love that surrounds them, and the memories that remain will comfort them, regardless of their beliefs.

70.   What response do you have for the person who asks, "How can I leave those I love?"

Do you believe you ever really leave? Reflections at life's end usually are not of the possessions acquired, the wealth, or home, or status, for these are not the most difficult to leave. It is the human, intimate connections that one cannot bear to lose. No matter how hard it may be to believe, it is true that when life for this body ends and the soul moves on, connection remains in the hearts of others, and the soul also carries awareness in connection with these people. Returning to a unified Source, as all are connected to this Source, the vibrations continue to relate to one another across time, space and other dimensions. The reason the question remains is that it is very difficult when living in body to imagine existing in other realms. To have consciousness outside this body seems inconceivable, and yet it is the message of faith that consciousness remains, even after the body is gone. So, to summarize the answer to "How can I leave that to which I am so attached?", you are not leaving but transforming the connection, and in transforming the connection, increasing the opportunity for growth for all who are present, and all who will meet again in later times.

On Faith and Understanding

Reason is a powerful tool, useful throughout life in a range of situations, but reason fails to explain the unexplainable, or to provide comfort when seeking to understand that which is beyond sight.

We speak now of faith and understanding, not knowledge based on logic and evidence, but the sure sweet certainty of knowing that mystery exists and the divine gift of eternal life is present for all. It is faith that allows for this certainty to grow and flower within, providing comfort and even serenity in life's most difficult passages. Yet the question is often asked, "How do I develop faith if I don't already have it?" Begin small, seek awareness of the tiniest of God's miracles and lost in the wonder of this awareness, allow yourself to feel the loving connection that surrounds you. Even in your most difficult moments simply close your eyes, let yourself desire support, and it is present. We are always available, but many feel that if they have not acknowledged mystery and powers beyond them when life has gone well, it is inappropriate to seek support in life's most painful passages. Be assured that we are grateful for the opportunity to serve and support. We wish to share both the way and your burden. With God's blessings, may all be pilgrims together.

The sun rises, but hope does not always join to greet the new day. Make full effort with awareness for the outcome is far less important than any can imagine.

CHAPTER XIII

WISHING FOR DEATH

Even though many fear death and seek to avoid it as long as possible, there may come a time when death seems desirable. Certainly this can occur for the aged, physically failing person. For those who stand helplessly by observing the suffering of those they love, there may be a wish as well for their parent's final release through death, for this, too, is a form of healing.

71.   Some people await death while others choose it. What can be said about suicide?

Both choices are equally valid. It is not whether one chooses to let life run its course, or chooses to end their life before their body chooses to end it that is most important. Rather, it is the process through which the decision is reached. The questions to be answered are, "Do I choose this consciously? Am I making this decision from an awareness of my soul's position, from an awareness of the impact this will have on the myriad of others who love me, or am I making this decision unconsciously?"

It is possible to extend your life to great lengths and remain unconscious, and it is possible to mindfully suicide. It is each individual's path to explore and right to decide this most significant issue.

72.   What is the burden placed on the soul of a decision of suicide?

In reality there are many passages to God's heaven, and if suicide is the passage that is chosen, then so be it. There is no unitary judgment that is imposed for any action. If one is mindful in their choices, they are choosing out of the most sincere belief that what they are doing is right for them. One can ask no more in this life than to choose well for oneself. Eventually, the soul will learn what is to be learned from this choice.

73.   You said it is possible to extend life. What do you mean?

Those who cry, "Just give me some time, time so that I may see a grandchild born", or time for some other heart's event, often find that time granted. This does not come from any external source, but rests in the individual's desire to cling to life. When this is no longer essential, letting go occurs. It is an opportunity for awareness that no matter what, some level of control rests within the individual.

74.   How do we bring comfort to those who watch a loved one fail, see the pain, and wish for that person's death?

Each person's path to self-acceptance will vary. Sometimes it is compassion for those who are dying that causes the greatest anguish. This anguish can be intensified by imagining themselves in the same position, and knowing they would wish for death under similar circumstances. There is nothing wrong in wishing that a person's suffering be diminished or ended. However, no individual can decide for another what the limit of their suffering is or should be, nor can they determine their wishes for them. This is an individual contract between each soul and God, and can only be witnessed and supported by others. When the time is done and the individual is ready, they leave, regardless of the wishes of those around them.

In the Stillness

The next time anxiety threatens to overtake the compassion within you, it is suggested that you sit quietly with these thoughts:

Continue and be aware.

Action is often most powerful
in your stillness.

Understanding is preceded by confusion,
just as love often follows the time of
your greatest emptiness.

Let your heart guide you and carry you
through these difficult times.

CHAPTER XIV

CONSCIOUSLY DYING

The approach of death may be ignored or denied as long as possible by the dying and their loved ones. That is one path. Another path is that of awareness, referred to as consciously dying. Here all denial is abandoned, and words like death and dying are embraced as a part of life, just as are birth and creation.

75. **Some people withdraw from life's daily activities. Are they engaged in consciously dying?**

The first question is whether this is really withdrawal, or rather a turning inward for reflection, reconciliation with self, and letting go of the extraneous. If the inward movement leads to an awareness of self, there is nothing wrong with lack of attachment to the external. There can even be an advantage to the loss of acuity of hearing, vision, and the loss of energy. Distractions become fewer and fewer, and towards the very end there is usually an expanded awareness in each moment as it drifts slowly by.

For the family and loved ones, this is often seen as letting go, depression, unhappiness, or a rejection of the love and compassion that is being offered. In no way need this be true. Certainly it is not automatic that when a person withdraws they are doing soul's work, but quite often at the end of life this is precisely what is happening. At this time, there is far more energy expended in the spiritual world than in the material world. The very end stage of life can be the best meditation on being in the moment. Each moment can develop a luminous quality of awareness. The fewer the stimuli, the fewer the distractions, the greater the opportunity to be in the full glory of the moment.

76.   When we see the elderly spending so many hours seemingly oblivious to their surroundings, what is really occurring?

This might best be described as talking with angels, being in a state where they can feel and experience other realities, but not necessarily communicate this to you. It is the very loss of their attachment to this world which allows them the ease to enter other realms. It is also true that as the body begins to detach there is an unwinding and disengaging between soul and body. Eventually, the detachment is so great that the soul just slips away. There is nothing wrong or sad in this, for it is the natural ending of the relationship between this soul and the body that has carried it.

**77.   The dying person may achieve a
measure of peace, but what of family
members who feel cheated by an end
that does not bring closure or
consolation for their own turbulent
emotions?**

First, all bitter fruit must be eliminated. Do not
accept it as an obligation to carry unpleasant history
forward. There is a great difference between wishing for
something that does not come, and allowing the failure
of that wish to carry through to the rest of your life. Do
not continually feel that what you needed most was
denied to you even at death. Freed of these painful bonds,
you can seek warmth, affection, and all of those qualities
you hoped to get from your parent from others instead.
Do not perpetuate the frustrations and pain that
characterized your relationship, but rather remain open
to a new way of being. If you refuse to see change, you
will continue to suffer from the same circumstances that
befell you with your parent. Do not permit abuse by the
parent to continue from beyond the grave. Most
importantly, remember this change is totally within your
own control.

An Exercise on Being Present in Dying

There is nothing unique in dying. What may be unique is consciously engaging death, rather than fearing it. An environment where consciousness is not repeatedly broken, and where it is respected, is helpful, for it is difficult to maintain attention and awareness, even intermittently, when being pulled, confused and otherwise taken away from awareness. Remain focused on your intent. It might be helpful to have someone read passages that are important to you, that have meaning at this time. If you are comfortable with a spiritual tradition, hearing the words of sages and teachers can be very helpful. Surround yourself with those who are close to you and will pray with you, if that is of comfort. Create a holy space for moment to moment awareness. Converse with the powers that guided and supported you throughout your life. If there is one person who provides you with special comfort and has the courage to bear witness with you, ask them to guide, reassure, and encourage you through this process of growing awareness. There is no single path. Let each seek safe passage in their own way.

CHAPTER XV

MOURNING

Anticipating death is painful, but in some ways it is kinder than unexpected death. It grants the time for reconciliation and loving connection, and begins the mourning process in a gentler way. At different stages of life, people may mourn differently. For example, a young adult may pass quickly through mourning, buoyed with the hope of the world that awaits their youth, but to a spouse of many years, death can be a time of despair and hopelessness. Mourning is a journey, like many others, and an evolution from direct connection to memory.

78.   What can be said about the mourning process that will help the bereaved?

Initially, the grey veil of sadness may cover all that exists, and everything is seen through the experience of the recent death. At the same time, it is a quieting period, an opportunity for internal reflection, for renewal and remembrance, a special time, in which remembering is necessary for completion. It is time to direct your attention inward, not so much in the immediate aftermath of the death and the funeral, but in the long weeks that follow, when gifts of food no longer arrive, and calls and visitors become less frequent. Use this time as an opportunity to reminisce, to reflect, to look at things done and not done and create a balance in your world when balance seems to have been lost. Be open to self discovery and you will emerge with greater strength and resources.

Although your loss is experienced, it can be integrated as you move forward. Loss is part of the great awakening of each individual to the knowledge that even as there is emptiness, there is relief; that even as you may feel very saddened by the loss, there are other events that can make you smile; that the world is full of a mix of experiences, and moment to moment your mood and reactions will change.

79.   Please discuss the varying impact of the death of a loved one.

Death is experienced in many ways by the survivors. The reactions vary widely from individual to individual, depending not just on their age, but also on their attachment to the person who has died and the implications of this death for them and their world. As to age, contrary to popular thinking, death can be very real for a child, and almost a fantasy for those adults who deny death.

There are some losses of such magnitude and such overwhelming impact that the individual will not recover in this lifetime from the loss. Such is the loss a small child experiences when their parent dies while the child is very young. Even though they are young and resilient, the two year old will never really heal from the loss of the mother or father at this stage. It is indeed a tear in the fabric of their soul, and the child will spend much of this lifetime trying to find the solace and comfort denied them as a consequence of their parent's death in these early years.

Mourning also relates to the nature of the loss, the circumstances, and whether those who remain feel strong or powerless. If the emotional needs of the mourner are met, the process of saying good bye is honored and the mourners can move on. It is extremely important that mourners complete leavetaking in a way that is of value to them. For a small child, it may be floating a boat on a pond in recognition of the transition of their loved one, or writing a letter and placing it in the casket, or reciting a prayer as they go to sleep. There are many different ways in which you can complete your role in mourning and be consoled.

Whatever method is used you discover that as time goes by, the heart becomes lighter and sad reflection and reminiscence diminish. More time will gradually be spent looking forward rather than backward. All of this is a valuable learning opportunity, for even as you mourn, recognize this is your work of the moment. Your prayers are received and accepted, and your thoughts fly to your loved one as prayers did the day they were buried.

It might be helpful for you to keep some note of your evolution through bereavement. Jot down your thoughts in the form of a diary or journal, or set aside some part of each day to reflect on yourself and on your life and the part the person, now dead, played in your world. Create something living and beautiful, for even tending a plant can connect you with life. Above all, allow yourself to be involved in life.

80.   What about the pain at the premature death of a loved one?

Death out of time is especially painful and it brings up feelings of helplessness, of hopes unrealized and even failure. It is very painful to lose someone who is young, but in the midst of the anguish are also issues of ego. With the death of a child the parent loses an extension of themselves, and someone they may have seen as their future, or even their immortality. The early death of a mate can leave the survivor adrift, unsure of their future, and of their identity. To reflect on how much of the pain is for the loss of the loved one and how much is sorrow for the loss of the future might be helpful, but it does not diminish the anguish of the mourner's suffering. The person who sees their loved one's life as a brief but wonderful gift will know greater peace and serenity in this troubled time. For those who see it only as a loss, and even a punishment, there is no solace.

Loss can be intense and profound, but the sheer aching of the loss is a reminder of all that is still present. Just as those who have lost a limb rarely stop feeling the

sensation of its presence, those who have lost a loved one
may be more keenly aware of the absence than they were
of the presence. This awareness can be transformed into
something of use and value, such as greater spiritual
understanding for themselves and others. Many difficult
lessons occur around loss and death. Without dismissing
the pain that is involved under all circumstances, the
suffering quite often is magnified by the individual's
unwillingness to see the possibility to move through and
transform this process.

An Exercise in Awareness

Mourning is a holy time, a time of ending, but also of awakening, a time of letting go of someone you love and a good time to reflect on all that you are and all that you wish to be.

Let us suggest an exercise in these extraordinary times. First, sit quietly and see before you your headstone. Let the words of the inscription emerge in your mind's eye. Do not be afraid to spend time in this space for God is with you, now as always. As these words enter your heart and your mind they will fill you with the essence of your life as it is best expressed. Sit with this, then take paper and pen and write those words that you hope will be spoken at your own funeral. Allow your heart to lead and let yourself expand into this new awareness. When you have completed this task, rest quietly and then read your words aloud. As your feelings emerge capture the best of them, and with God's guidance shape your future. Accept the opportunity of this moment to create your life anew, so that each step is in the light of the Path you have chosen. With God's grace, travel on.

CHAPTER XVI

FUNERAL RITES

Funerals are an old tradition of celebration, a way
of designating a passage from one form to another. They
are both practical and transcendental, and their import is
great. Unfortunately, the spiritual aspect is often
minimized and sanitized to the point of uselessness in
today's world. This is unwise for both body and spirit, for
in a world where little outside the mundane is ritualized,
funerals remain one of the few passages noted. Their
importance remains constant, although often modified
across time to be more in keeping with the material
world.

**81. What part do funerals and rituals play
      in life's drama?**

A culture or religious group may be defined by its
burial tradition and its manner of dealing with both
dying and death. Years ago when one died, the body
would rest in the home, surrounded by loved ones, with

candles lit, creating an atmosphere conducive to reflection. It was a time for grief and the beginning of healing. Today, however, circumstances are quite different, and most often your loved one dies in a cold and sterile place separate from family, carried away to a funeral home where they are embalmed, made to look like something they had not been, and displayed for at least the immediate family. Rather than a meaningful ritual, this can become a social event, a status statement speaking to the devotion of the family. Do you really believe that the soul's way is sped by a mahogany casket? Do you honestly believe that one cannot change form and move as spirit without being dressed in a really fine suit?

This change of custom from past to present occurred gradually and insidiously. Once the discomfort was removed, the funeral process became as comfortable and familiar as buying new furnishings for your home. Ideally, the funeral is a place apart, an opportunity to reflect, to give passage, to mourn, and find peace. It functions as a gathering together of many who care, a sharing, a united voice of prayer where the individual is wished well on their way, and the family, experiencing this death as a great loss, is supported.

All you need as your loved one is laid to rest is this advice.

Simple words seek the skies.

Complicated thoughts are not required.

Let the prayers rise like smoke to the heavens,

And be observed by the angels who await.

**82.   Funerals also provide a statement
for the family. The costly casket
symbolizes that this person was special.
What harm is there in that?**

While not automatically detrimental, it is still a
diversion. Spending large sums on an elaborate funeral is
merely being material where emphasis should be on a
spiritual transition. If, additionally, material display is
done out of a sense of guilt or out of a desire to presume
status, no lasting comfort will be found.

If one wishes to provide a glorious memory of the
individual who has passed on, the money can be offered
to charity, as a loving recognition of that person's
values, rather than burying it beneath the ground. This
can be broadly interpreted and need not be limited to
major charities, but serves to express the essence of the
person who has died. Understand that the wish here is
not to deny people the comfort of display, but to remind
them that this is a spiritual transition.

**83.   What about the funeral as a statement
to the community by the family
showing how much the departed was
valued?**

It is difficult to see into the hearts of mourners and
understand their concern with what others might think of
them. Loved ones are valued in the hearts of those who
care. In the process of elaborate funeral arrangements,
more attention may be placed on the status of the

survivors than on the valued qualities of the departed. We wish great peace and relief from suffering for those who mourn, but it is of less concern whether their neighbors are impressed. If there is a desire to have status in the eyes of the community, there are many ways in which memorials can be offered. Let those be examined and offered, each within the keeping of your own heart. It is not about money, but about continuing the memory in the manner of the individual who has died. An elaborate funeral does not create the continuity you may desire. A far greater memorial would be to spend an hour a week in a nursing home befriending those who have no visitors, than to buy the casket, or the headstone, or even the plaque. Remember, too, that the stranger in the nursing home is no stranger, but someone you have not yet had the opportunity to know in this lifetime. Souls spring from one Source and all are connected. What is required is the extension of human compassion, as opposed to further activity in a material world.

The personal impact of your loss is great, but only by dealing directly with that loss, and permitting that person to live on in spirit, is the real work of the mourning process completed.

84.   Please speak to us about cremation.

Each method of dealing with the body that has dropped is valuable or not, depending on the perspective of those observing it. Such things vary by custom, community, social habit, and the practical need for dealing with flesh which is no longer sustained by the soul's fire. There is nothing either right or wrong with burial or cremation, or, in fact, any of the myriad ways in which bodies are offered back to the earth. The difficulty is assuming that your path is the only path. Look to your heart and discover what matters most for you as an individual, and for those you love. This is an emotionally charged issue, and one which could lead to many productive conversations about "Who am I? What am I? What aspects of me have value and matter?"

85.   When people gather after the funeral or cremation, there is sometimes an atmosphere of laughter and hilarity. Is this appropriate?

It is just and fit that even in death life goes on. Laughter is not a saintly thing, but uniquely human, and the ability to be amused at anything is very much a consequence of the human brain, and its capacity to put thoughts together in unusual and novel ways. It is good to remember the absurdity and frailties of the human form at this time, as well as other times. Any chance to smile and grasp at amusement during these times can result in joyous and warm remembrance. Do not take yourself too seriously, for the overblown ego loses its humor, and healing often begins with humor. On a pragmatic level, humor is a way of easing tension and distracting the mourners. Of course, laughter that is excessive, raucous, or cruel can be especially painful to the newly bereaved. It is for each to decide what is appropriate at this time.

It is not what you expected, but the vantage is one which affords you great wisdom. The world creates and recreates in each living thing and all are of equal importance and wonder.

CHAPTER XVII

THE TRANSITION

It is interesting that when people think of aging and debilitation, they think of a dark tunnel, but as they actually approach death and enter the dying process, they find themselves in a tunnel of light. Here as elsewhere, light and dark are a matter of perspective. When you are fully engaged in the process of leaving, it feels like one candle after another is being snuffed out. With the realization that the body is something to be left behind, you finally look forward and see the light of a thousand candles beckoning you.

86.   When death is imminent, part of the fear is that all communication will end and there will be no further connection. Please speak to this concern.

For most, the awareness that they are about to die is painful. It is seen as an abrupt separation from all that is known and loved. Initially it is experienced as entering into a terrifying darkness, and only later becomes a gentle walk to a brighter reality. Living in a rational world, it is difficult to imagine that spirits can communicate, but it is true in the sense of awareness, in the sense of presence, and in the form of memories and recollections. As an individual enters the final stages of life review and prepares to die, they begin to experience attention from those hovering just beyond in another dimension. It is these spirits who will guide and support them in their journey onward. With time, the dying become more willing and aware of the gentle support of these spirits, and slowly relax into the transition. The realization that spirits await to ease their passage leads to the understanding that they, too, will be available to those they leave behind. This is not to say that there is no shift in the nature of relationships, for survivors may be very caught up in grieving, and feeling the loss of the physical presence of those who have died. And yet, the individual who has changed form and gone to another plane will be fully available to enter into the process of connection.

87.   Many people who have suffered the loss of a loved one have tried to make this connection without success. Would you speak to this?

The difficulty often is not in reaching someone who has moved to another dimension, but the expectation that they appear or connect in a specific manner. In other words, "They are not here unless I see them, feel them touch my arm, and are dressed as they have always been." In fact, it is extremely easy to contact those who have come and gone, just as it is easy to contact another who is in this world in this time and space. For instance, you have many friends and family surrounding you, across this country, and even in other lands. While thinking of them send your thoughts onward, and they will receive them. Even as you go through your day you may find yourself saying, "Ah! I am thinking of someone I have not thought of for some time. Maybe I will call them." And, sure enough, if you were to examine this and take it back to that friend who is at some distance, you would find that a connection was happening at that time. How many times have you called someone and they have responded, "I was just thinking about you." Just as it can happen on earth when all are living, so it can happen across lifetimes.

88. **It also happens that you are thinking of someone, sure that you are making a connection, but if you follow it up you discover the other person was oblivious to your efforts. It leads one to distrust the possibility of connection.**

You do not distrust the telephone. When you pick up the phone to call someone, there is no guarantee they will be there to answer your call, but that does not make you believe the telephone is an invalid instrument. It merely causes you to think they are out of that space at that time, or not currently accepting phone calls. So it is with transmissions of thought or feeling. There is required a mutual receptivity, for it is not enough to merely offer the thought.

89.   Are the deceased close after death?

It is as if the living and those who have died travel on parallel roads just far enough distant to be obscured one from the other. Ultimately, the roads turn in separate directions as each follows his own way, but initially, both monitor the same events, and address the same issues.

90.   Are they able to make their presence known to their loved ones?

This is always possible and there are many such instances. Some spirits will attempt connection, some will not, some loved ones will notice, and some will not. There is always the possibility for beings to touch back, and at this time, shortly after death, contact is often easiest. However, it is not in the best interest of the soul who has left, or even those who remain, to have much contact at this point. Do not hold people's spirits in attachment to the earth, but allow the souls to move forward. They have much work to do on their plane, just as the living have work to do on this plane.

Meeting in Dreams

My grandfather had always been there for me when I was a small child. Warm, supportive and filled with stories, he was my safe haven in a complicated world. All his grandchildren loved him and there was great sadness when he died in my tenth year. As time passed, the memories remained, but the pain diminished. I will never forget his love. One night, while I slept in the dormitory at my college, I had a dream. In this dream my grandfather appeared looking much as he had always looked. Although he did not speak, I was filled with the warmth of his love and support. He looked happy and peaceful, fully connected, yet clearly elsewhere. I awoke from my night's sleep rested and fondly remembered the dream.

Two weeks later I was speaking with my sister, Sarah, and mentioned my dream in passing. Surprised, she responded that she had the same dream. We then realized he had come to both of us on the same night. We both knew that he had come to reassure us and wish us well. We knew he was at peace, and now we are at peace as well.

It is time for the work to begin, dreaming finished, movement and action required. Let no fears stand in your way, but move with the certainty of momentum, the confidence of your own future.

CHAPTER XVIII

CONCLUSION

Like a stream that has traveled along the mountainside for a great distance, you have arrived at the end of this reading. The rushing mountain torrent has become smaller and more gentle. Now it forms an almost still pool at the base of the mountain, a place for reflection in depth, awareness and quiet contemplation. All that need be said has been said, but this is a fitting time to reflect, review, and gather in all that has been gained in this journey. Let us review what has been discovered.

First, suffering, pain and the difficulties of aging and loss, are opportunities for discovery offered you in this world. Painful as they may be, often tedious and draining they provide an opportunity to move forward in understanding of yourself, and in relation to the plan that is this universe. Exploring the many aspects of the changes that come at the end of life, but not the end of time, you let go one after the other of attachments, which however compelling, are merely temporary. These attachments, lovingly held in their time, are released as the need for them diminishes. First to be released is the material, and the many expectations of body and mind. As the world and all that it carries within it for you grows more distant and more simplified, your luminous soul emerges. It is this emergence, the re-emergence of the beauty that came into the body at birth, that explains why the process of ending is truly a beginning. This is so for the person who is leaving, and for those who love and are connected to them, as they move together on the wheel of time.

On the material level, little is left when all else is gone, when neither strength, nor health, nor possessions in most cases, remain. Only the body is left. But that part which is held most dear, and is in fact the enduring you, has been only temporarily housed in these trappings which are falling away. The soul has journeyed, offered much in gaining much, developed brightness and inner wisdom in this lifetime. As it slips out of the form that no longer sustains it, the soul is free to move elsewhere, to a free-of-body awareness and consciousness, a return to the Light, joining with the energy of all that is, all that ever was, and all that ever shall be. And yet for those resting on this plane, it is hard to see the other side. Both exist, but depending on your perspective one may have far greater reality than the other. It might be wise to remember that it is not the destination that is important, but the experience of the journey, and all that one learns and discovers and offers on the tour they have taken on this planet in this lifetime.

Life is a deep and abiding reflection on the meaningfulness of impermanence and change, and the value of letting go. You develop grace and wisdom in the process of seeing the true person, as opposed to the fiction created through physical and material means. It is this stripping away that is the work of great age. It is a wonderful, final opportunity for the person who is letting go, and it is even more an opportunity for those who care to participate in the process of helping a soul free itself from attachments. As the true self breaks free of old habits, old memories, and, in fact, all the old aspects carried for many years, there is a lighter quality. They may seem more playful, more luminous, and in some ways far freer than they have been. This is the pure essence that is released when the body is dropped.

Much has been said and explored in this book, but words are merely words unless experienced and brought into the heart. As important as these lessons are, they are not to be read, but to be lived. Work with chapters as lessons to be explored. Meditate and review. Expand your awareness as your heart opens to this task, and let the work conform to your needs at this time. For those of you who are caregivers, reflect on the aspects most relevant to caregiving. For those who struggle with the dementia of a loved one, let your awareness be shaped and your consciousness expand in that regard. Remember that you are not alone or unsupported in this journey, but are part of a larger plan to bring all to awareness, peace, and ultimately, comfort in the Light.

Capture the art of falling into your understanding as well as striving towards it. Surrender and search are both necessary.

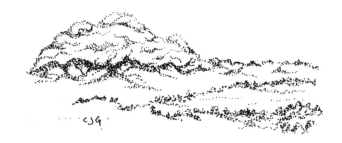

Dear Readers,

We hope you have enjoyed this book and that it provided you with insights that will prove valuable. We have been told by other readers that they, too, had stories to tell that were relevant to the issues addressed in **Decisions to Make, Paths to Take.**

We invite you to share your stories with us and would be pleased to hear from you. Please send all correspondence to us at:

Decision Press
P.O. Box 741254
Boynton Beach, FL 33474-1254

We will respond to all letters and look forward to your personal stories.

Sincerely,

Joy Pelzmann & Myrna Rosoff

Resources

Alzheimer's Disease & Related Disorder Association
919 Michigan Ave.
Suite 1000
Chicago, IL 60611
800-272-3900
Information and referrals on dementia

American Association of Homes and Services for the Aging
901 E St., N.W.
Suite 500
Washington, D.C. 20004
Care-giving brochures

American Association of Retired Persons (AARP)
601 E St., N.W.
Washington, D.C. 20049
202-434-2277
Free publications on all aspects of elder affairs and care

Center for Books on Aging
1331 H St., N.W.
Washington, D.C. 20005
800-221-4272
Catalog of books and tapes on aging

Children of Aging Parents
     Woodbourne Office Campus
     Suite 302A
     1809 Woodbourne Rd.
     Levittown, PA 19057
          212-945-6900
          Comprehensive information resources

Choice in Dying
     200 Varick St.
     New York, N.Y. 10014
          800-989-9455
          Legal forms for health care directives

For your County's Department (or Division) of Aging:
     Check local telephone book under Government-
     Human Services or Social Services

Foundation for Hospice & Home Care
     320 A St., N.E.
     Washington, D.C. 20002
          202-547-6586
          Information and referrals

Funeral & Memorial Societies of America
6900 Lost Lake Rd.
Egg Harbor, WI 54209
800-765-0107
Information on inexpensive services

National Association of Area Agencies on Aging
1112 16th St., N.W.
Suite 100
Washington, D.C. 20036
800-677-1116 Eldercare Locator Service
Referrals to community assistance for
seniors

National Cancer Institute
Building 31, Room 10A24
Bethesda, MD 20892
800-422-6237
Information and referrals to local groups

National Associations for specific diseases, such as
Alzheimer's, Cancer, Heart,
Diabetes, Parkinson's, Stroke
Check local telephone book

National Council on Aging
409 3rd St., S.W.
Suite 200
Washington, D.C. 20024
800-424-9046
Referrals to local service agencies, free
pamphlet

National Family Caregivers Association
9621 E. Bexhill Dr.
Kensington, MD 20895-3104
800-535-3198
http://www.nfacares.org
Support network, newsletter

National Hospice Organization
1901 N. Moore St.
Suite 901
Arlington, VA 22209
800-658-8898
Information about care for the
terminally ill

Nursing Home Information Center
1331 F St., N.W.
Washington, D.C. 20004-1171
202-347-8800
Information and referrals for
long-term services

For your State's Department (or Division) of Aging:
Check the telephone book for the state capitol

State Motor Vehicle Division for problems persuading
unsafe drivers to give up driving

U.S. Department of Veteran's Affairs
Check local telephone book
Comprehensive care and services for veterans

ORDER FORM

DECISIONS TO MAKE, PATHS TO TAKE

Name_____

Address_____

City_____State_____Zip_____

No. of copies____@ $13.95   Subtotal: $_____

Plus postage & handling (per book)

      1st Class $3.50 per book $_____

      Book Rate $2.50 per book $_____

(Maximum postage for multiple orders: $10.00)

Florida Residents add 6% Sales Tax $_____

                  Total: $_____

Send check or money order to:

   DECISION PRESS
   P.O. Box 741254
   Boynton Beach, FL 33474-1254
   or call (561) 731-0064

NOTES

NOTES

NOTES

ORDER FORM

DECISIONS TO MAKE, PATHS TO TAKE

Name_____

Address_____

City_____State_____Zip_____

No. of copies____@ $13.95   Subtotal: $_____

Plus postage & handling (per book)

   1st Class $3.50 per book $_____

   Book Rate $2.50 per book $_____

(Maximum postage for multiple orders: $10.00)

Florida Residents add 6% Sales Tax $_____

        Total: $_____

Send check or money order to:

 DECISION PRESS
 P.O. Box 741254
 Boynton Beach, FL 33474-1254
 or call (561) 731-0064